QuickFACTS™

From the Experts at the American Cancer Society

Prostate CANCER

What You Need to Know—NOW

SECOND EDITION

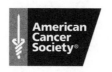

Published by the American Cancer Society/Health Promotions
250 Williams Street NW, Atlanta, Georgia 30303 USA

Copyright ©2011 American Cancer Society

Printed in the United States of America
Cover designed by Jill Dible, Atlanta, GA
Composition by Graphic Composition, Inc.

5 4 3 2 1   11 12 13 14 15

Library of Congress Cataloging-in-Publication Data

Quickfacts prostate cancer: what you need to know-now / from the experts at the American Cancer Society. — 2nd ed.
    p. cm. — (Quick facts)
   Includes bibliographical references and index.
   ISBN-13: 978-1-60443-008-0 (pbk. : alk. paper)
   ISBN-10: 1-60443-008-7 (pbk. : alk. paper)
   1. Prostate—Cancer—Popular works. I. American Cancer Society. II. Title: Prostate cancer
   RC280.P7Q53 2011
   616.99'463–dc22

                    2010017109

A Note to the Reader

This information represents the views of the doctors and nurses serving on the American Cancer Society's Cancer Information Database Editorial Board. These views are based on their interpretation of studies published in medical journals, as well as their own professional experience.

The treatment information in this book is not official policy of the Society and is not intended as medical advice to replace the expertise and judgment of your cancer care team. It is intended to help you and your family make informed decisions, together with your doctor.

Your doctor may have reasons for suggesting a treatment plan different from these general treatment options. Don't hesitate to ask him or her questions about your treatment options.

For more information, contact your American Cancer Society at **800-227-2345** or **cancer.org**.

Bulk purchases of this book are available at a discount. For information, contact the American Cancer Society at **trade.sales@cancer.org**.

For special sales, contact us at **trade.sales@cancer.org**.

*Quick*FACTS™

Prostate
CANCER

What You Need to Know — NOW

TABLE OF CONTENTS

Considering Prostate Cancer Treatment Options

Questions to Ask

After Treatment

Your Prostate Cancer

What Is Cancer?

The body is made up of hundreds of millions of living **cells**.* Normal body cells grow, divide, and die in an orderly fashion. During the early years of a person's life, normal cells divide faster to allow the person to grow. After the person becomes an adult, most cells divide only to replace worn-out or dying cells or to repair injuries.

Cancer begins when cells in a part of the body start to grow out of control. There are many kinds of cancer, but they all start because of out-of-control growth of abnormal cells.

Cancer cell growth is different from normal cell growth. Instead of dying, **cancer cells** continue to grow and form new, abnormal cells. Cancer cells can also invade (grow into) other tissues, something that normal cells cannot do. Growing out of control and invading other tissues are what makes a cell a cancer cell.

Cells become cancer cells because of damage to **DNA**. DNA is in every cell and directs all its

*Terms in **bold type** are further explained in the Glossary, beginning on page 171.

actions. In a normal cell, when DNA gets damaged the cell either repairs the damage or the cell dies. In cancer cells, the damaged DNA is not repaired, but the cell doesn't die like it should. Instead, this cell goes on making new cells that the body does not need. These new cells will all have the same damaged DNA as the first cell does.

People can inherit damaged DNA, but most DNA damage is caused by mistakes that happen while the normal cell is reproducing or by something in our environment. Sometimes the cause of the DNA damage is something obvious, like cigarette smoking. But often no clear cause is found.

In most cases, the cancer cells form a **tumor**. Some cancers, like leukemia, rarely form tumors. Instead, these cancer cells involve the blood and blood-forming organs and circulate through other tissues where they grow.

Cancer cells often travel to other parts of the body, where they begin to grow and form new tumors that replace normal **tissue**. This process is called **metastasis**. It happens when the cancer cells get into the bloodstream or lymph vessels of our body.

No matter where a cancer may spread, it is always named for the place where it started. For example, breast cancer that has spread to the liver is still called breast cancer, not liver cancer. Likewise, prostate cancer that has spread to the bone is **metastatic** prostate cancer, not bone cancer.

Different types of cancer can behave very differently. For example, lung cancer and breast cancer are very different diseases. They grow at different rates and respond to different treatments. That is why people with cancer need treatment that is aimed at their particular kind of cancer.

Not all tumors are **malignant** (cancerous). Tumors that aren't cancer are called **benign**. Benign tumors can cause problems—they can grow very large and press on healthy organs and tissues. But they cannot invade (grow into) other tissues. Because they can't invade, they also can't **metastasize** (spread) to other parts of the body. These tumors are almost never life threatening.

What Is Prostate Cancer?

About the Prostate

The **prostate** is a walnut-sized **gland** located in front of the **rectum** and underneath the urinary **bladder**. It is found only in men. The prostate's job is to make some of the fluid that protects and nourishes sperm cells in semen. Just behind the prostate gland are the **seminal vesicles** that make most of the fluid for semen. The **urethra**, which is the tube that carries urine and semen out of the body through the penis, runs through the prostate.

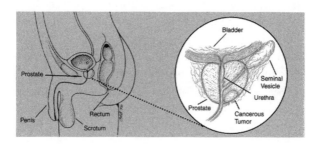

The prostate starts to develop before birth and continues to grow until a man reaches adulthood. This growth is fueled by male **hormones** (called **androgens**) in the body. The main androgen, **testosterone**, is made in the **testicles**. The enzyme **5 alpha-reductase** converts testosterone into **dihydrotestosterone (DHT)**. DHT signals the prostate to grow. The prostate stays at adult size in adults as long as male hormones are present. In older men, the inner part of the prostate (around the urethra) often keeps growing, leading to a common condition called **benign prostatic hyperplasia (BPH)**. In BPH, the prostate tissue can press on the urethra, leading to problems passing urine. Although BPH can be a serious medical problem, it is not cancer.

Prostate Cancer

Several types of cells are found in the prostate, but more than 99% of prostate cancers develop from the gland cells. Gland cells make the prostate fluid that is added to the semen. The medical term for a cancer that starts in gland cells is **adenocarcinoma**.

Other types of cancer can also start in the prostate gland, including sarcomas, small cell carcinomas, and transitional cell carcinomas. But because these other types of prostate cancer are so rare, if you have prostate cancer it is almost certain to be an adenocarcinoma. *The rest of this book refers only to prostate adenocarcinoma.*

Some prostate cancers can grow and spread quickly, but most of them grow slowly. In fact, autopsy studies show that many older men (and even some younger men) who died of other diseases also had prostate cancer that never affected them during their lives. In these studies, 70% to 90% of the men had cancer in their prostate by age 80, but in many cases neither they nor their doctors even knew they had it.

Precancerous Conditions of the Prostate

Many doctors believe that prostate cancer begins with a precancerous condition called **prostatic intraepithelial neoplasia (PIN)**. PIN begins to appear in the prostates of some men as early as their 20s. Almost half of all men have PIN by the time they reach 50. In this condition, there are changes in how the prostate gland cells look under the microscope, but the abnormal cells don't look like they are growing into other parts of the prostate (like cancer cells would). The cell changes are classified as either low grade, meaning the patterns of prostate cells appear almost normal, or high grade, meaning they look more abnormal.

If you have had high-grade PIN found on a prostate **biopsy**, there is about a 20% to 30% chance that you also have cancer in another area of your prostate. This is why doctors often watch men with high-grade PIN carefully and may advise a repeat prostate biopsy, especially if the original biopsy did not take samples from all parts of the prostate.

Another finding that may be reported on a prostate biopsy is **atypical small acinar proliferation (ASAP)**, which is sometimes just called **atypia**. In ASAP, the cells look like they might be cancerous when viewed under the microscope, but there are too few of them on the slide to be sure. If ASAP is found, there's about a 40% to 50% chance that cancer is also present in the prostate. This is why many doctors advise getting a repeat biopsy within a few months.

Another finding that may be reported on a prostate biopsy is **proliferative inflammatory atrophy (PIA)**. In PIA, the cells look abnormal when viewed under the microscope. PIA is not cancer, but researchers believe that some PIA cells can turn into prostate cancer directly or by first changing into high-grade PIN.

What Are the Key Statistics About Prostate Cancer?

Other than skin cancer, prostate cancer is the most common cancer in American men. The latest American Cancer Society estimates for prostate cancer in the United States are for 2010:

- About 217,730 new cases of prostate cancer will be diagnosed.
- About 32,050 men will die of prostate cancer.

About 1 man in 6 will receive a **diagnosis** of prostate cancer during his lifetime. More than 2 million men in the United States who have had prostate cancer at some point are still alive today.

Prostate cancer is the second leading cause of cancer death in American men, behind only lung cancer. About 1 man in 35 will die of prostate cancer. Prostate cancer accounts for about 10% of cancer-related deaths in men.

The **5-year survival rate** refers to the percentage of patients who live at least 5 years after their cancer is diagnosed. These rates are used to create a standard way of discussing **prognosis** (outlook). Of course, many of these patients live much longer than 5 years after diagnosis. Five-year survival rates are based on cancers diagnosed and first treated more than 5 years ago. Improvements in treatment since then may result in a better outlook for patients with recently diagnosed cancer. **Five-year relative survival rates** compare the observed survival with that expected for people without the cancer. That means that relative survival only talks about deaths from the cancer in question. This is a more accurate way to describe the outlook for patients with a certain cancer.

According to the most recent data, for all men with prostate cancer, the relative 5-year survival rate is nearly 100% and the relative 10-year survival rate is 91%. The 15-year relative survival rate is 76%. Keep in mind that 5-year survival rates are based on cancers diagnosed and first treated more than 5 years ago, and 10-year survival rates are based on cancers diagnosed more than 10 years ago. Modern methods of detection and treatment mean that many prostate cancers are now found earlier and can be treated more effectively. If you receive a diagnosis of prostate cancer this year, your outlook is likely to be better than the numbers reported above.

Risk Factors and Causes

What Are the Risk Factors for Prostate Cancer?

A **risk factor** is anything that affects your chance of getting a disease such as cancer. Different cancers have different risk factors. For example, exposing skin to strong sunlight is a risk factor for skin cancer. Smoking is a risk factor for many cancers.

But risk factors don't tell us everything. Many people with one or more risk factors never get cancer, while others who get cancer may have had no known risk factors.

We don't yet completely understand the causes of prostate cancer, but researchers have found several factors that may change the risk of getting it. For some of these factors, the link to prostate cancer risk is not yet clear.

Age

Age is the strongest risk factor for prostate cancer. Prostate cancer is very rare before the age of 40, but the chance of having prostate cancer rises rapidly after age 50. Almost 2 of 3 prostate cancers are found in men over the age of 65.

Race/Ethnicity

Prostate cancer occurs more often in black men than in men of other races. Black men are also more likely to receive a diagnosis of prostate cancer at an advanced stage, and are more than twice as likely to die of the disease than white men. Prostate cancer occurs less often in Asian American and Hispanic/Latino men than in non-Hispanic whites. The reasons for these racial and ethnic differences are not clear.

Nationality

Prostate cancer is most common in North America, northwestern Europe, Australia, and the Caribbean islands. It is less common in Asia, Africa, Central America, and South America. The reasons for this finding are not clear. More intensive **screening** in some developed countries likely accounts for at least part of this difference, but other factors are likely to be important as well. For example, lifestyle differences such as diet may be important: men of Asian descent living in the United States have a lower risk of prostate cancer than white Americans but a higher risk of prostate cancer than men of similar backgrounds living in Asia.

Family History

Prostate cancer seems to run in some families, which suggests that, in some cases, there may be an inherited or genetic factor. Having a father or brother with prostate cancer more than doubles a man's risk of developing this disease. (The risk is higher for men with an affected brother than for those with an affected father.) The risk is much higher for men with several affected relatives, particularly if their relatives were young at the time the cancer was found.

Genes

Scientists have found several inherited **genes** that seem to raise prostate cancer risk, but they probably account for only a small number of cases overall. Genetic testing for most of these genes is not yet available. Recently, some common gene variations have been linked to the risk of prostate cancer. Studies to confirm these results are needed to see if testing for the gene variants will be useful in predicting prostate cancer risk.

Some inherited genes raise the risk for more than one type of cancer. For example, inherited **mutations** of the **BRCA1** or **BRCA2** genes are the reason that breast and ovarian cancers are much more common in some families. Mutations in these genes may also increase prostate cancer risk in some men, but they account for a very small percentage of prostate cancer cases.

Diet

The exact role of diet in prostate cancer is not clear, but several different factors have been studied.

Men who eat a lot of red meat or high-fat dairy products appear to have a slightly higher chance of getting prostate cancer. These men also tend to eat fewer fruits and vegetables. Doctors are not sure which of these factors is responsible for raising the risk.

Some studies have suggested that men who consume a lot of calcium (through food or supplements) may be at higher risk for advanced prostate cancer. Most studies have not found such a link with the levels of calcium found in the average diet, and it is important to note that calcium is known to have other important health benefits.

Obesity

Most studies have not found that obesity (having a high amount of extra body fat) puts men at higher risk for prostate cancer. Some studies have found that obese men have a lower risk of getting a low-grade (less dangerous) form of the disease, but a higher risk of getting more aggressive prostate cancer. The reasons for this finding are not clear. Some studies have also found that obese men may be at greater risk for having more advanced prostate cancer and dying of prostate cancer, but this was not seen in other studies.

Exercise

Exercise has not been shown to reduce prostate cancer risk in most studies. But some studies have found that high levels of physical activity, particularly in older men, may lower the risk of advanced prostate cancer. More research in this area is needed.

Smoking

A recent study linked smoking to a small increase in the risk of death from prostate cancer. This is a new finding and will need to be confirmed by other studies.

Medicines

Some studies have found that men who took aspirin for many years had a lower risk of prostate cancer. At this time, however, taking aspirin to prevent prostate cancer is not recommended. Aspirin, even in low doses, can have serious side effects, including bleeding from the stomach. Also, the effect of aspirin on prostate cancer risk has only been studied by looking at men who were taking aspirin regularly for some other reason (like heart disease). This effect would need to be studied further before aspirin could be recommended as a way to prevent prostate cancer.

Recent studies have linked taking cholesterol-lowering drugs known as statins to a lower risk of advanced prostate cancer. This effect would need to be studied further before these drugs could be recommended as a way to prevent advanced prostate cancer.

The drugs finasteride and dutasteride have been shown to reduce the risk of prostate cancer in randomized, clinical trials. This is discussed in more detail in the section, "Can Prostate Cancer Be Prevented?" on pages 18–21.

Inflammation of the Prostate

Some studies have suggested that **prostatitis** (inflammation of the prostate gland) may be linked to an increased risk of prostate cancer, but other studies have not found such a link. Inflammation is often seen in samples of prostate tissue that also contain cancer. The link between the two is not yet clear, but this is an active area of research.

Infection

Researchers have also examined whether sexually transmitted infections (like gonorrhea or chlamydia) increase the risk of prostate cancer, possibly by leading to inflammation of the prostate. So far, studies have not agreed, and no firm conclusions have been reached.

Vasectomy

Some earlier studies suggested that men who had had a **vasectomy** (minor surgery to make men infertile)—especially those younger than 35 at the time of the procedure—were at a slightly increased risk for prostate cancer. But most recent studies have not found any increased risk among men who have had this operation. Fear of an increased risk of prostate cancer should not be a reason to avoid a vasectomy.

Prevention and Detection

Do We Know What Causes Prostate Cancer?

We still do not know exactly what causes prostate cancer. But researchers have found some risk factors and are trying to learn just how these factors cause prostate cells to become cancerous (see section, "What Are the Risk Factors for Prostate Cancer?").

On a basic level, prostate cancer is caused by changes in the DNA of a prostate cancer cell. During the past few years, scientists have made great progress in understanding how certain changes in DNA can cause normal prostate cells to grow abnormally and form cancers. DNA is the chemical that carries the instructions for nearly everything our cells do. The reason that you might look like your parents is because they are the source of your DNA.

DNA affects more than the way you look. Some genes (parts of your DNA) contain instructions for controlling when cells grow and divide. Certain genes that promote cell growth and division are called **oncogenes**. Others that normally slow down cell division or cause cells to die at the right time are called **tumor suppressor genes**. Cancer can be caused by DNA changes (mutations) that turn on oncogenes or turn off tumor suppressor genes.

DNA changes can either be inherited from a parent or can be acquired during a person's lifetime.

Inherited DNA Mutations

Researchers have found inherited DNA changes in certain genes may cause about 5% to 10% of prostate cancers.

Several mutated genes have been found that may be responsible for a man's inherited tendency for prostate cancer to develop. One of these is called **HPC1** (**H**ereditary **P**rostate **C**ancer Gene **1**). But there are many other gene mutations that may account for some cases of hereditary prostate cancer. None of these is a major cause, and more research on these genes is being done. Genetic tests are not yet available.

As mentioned above, men with BRCA1 or BRCA2 gene changes may be at an increased risk for prostate cancer. Mutations in these genes more commonly cause breast and ovarian cancer in women. But BRCA changes probably explain only a very small number of prostate cancers.

DNA Mutations Acquired During a Man's Lifetime

Most DNA mutations related to prostate cancer seem to develop during a man's life rather than having been inherited. Every time a cell prepares to divide into 2 new cells, it must copy its DNA. This process is not perfect, and sometimes errors occur, leaving the flawed DNA in the new cell.

It is not clear how many of these DNA mutations might be random events and how many may be influenced by other factors (diet, hormone levels, etc.). In general, the more quickly prostate cells grow and divide, the more chances there are for mutations to occur. Therefore, anything that speeds up this process may make prostate cancer more likely.

The development of prostate cancer may be linked to increased levels of certain hormones. High levels of androgens (male hormones, such as testosterone) promote prostate cell growth, and may contribute to prostate cancer risk in some men.

Some researchers have noted that men with high levels of another hormone, **insulin-like growth factor-1 (IGF-1)**, are more likely to get prostate cancer. IGF-1 hormone is similar to insulin, but it works on cell growth, not sugar metabolism. However, other studies have not found a link between IGF-1 and prostate cancer. Further research is needed to make sense of these findings.

As mentioned in the "What Are the Risk Factors for Prostate Cancer?" section on pages 9–14, some recent studies have found that inflammation may contribute to prostate cancer. One theory is that inflammation may lead to cell DNA damage, which might in turn push a cell closer to becoming cancerous. More research in this area is needed.

Exposure to radiation or cancer-causing chemicals may cause DNA mutations in many organs of the body, but these factors have not been proven to be important causes of mutations in prostate cells.

Can Prostate Cancer Be Prevented?

The exact cause of prostate cancer is not known, so at this time it is not possible to prevent most cases of the disease. Many risk factors such as age, race, and family history cannot be controlled. But based on what we do know, some cases might be prevented.

Diet

You may be able to reduce your risk of prostate cancer by changing the way you eat, but the results of research studies are not yet clear.

The American Cancer Society recommends choosing foods and beverages in amounts that help achieve and maintain a healthy weight, eating a variety of healthful foods with an emphasis on plant sources, and limiting your intake of red meats, especially high-fat or processed meats. Eat 5 or more servings of fruits and vegetables each day. Whole-grain breads, cereals, rice, pasta, and beans are also recommended. These guidelines on nutrition may also lower the risk for some other types of cancer, as well as other health problems.

Tomatoes (raw, cooked, or in tomato products such as sauces or ketchup), pink grapefruit, and watermelon are rich in **lycopenes**. These vitamin-like substances are antioxidants that help prevent damage to DNA. Some earlier studies suggested that lycopenes may help lower prostate cancer risk, but a more recent study found no link between blood levels of lycopene and risk of prostate cancer. Research in this area continues.

Vitamin and Mineral Supplements

There has been hope for some time that taking vitamin or mineral supplements might affect prostate cancer risk. Some studies have suggested that taking vitamin E daily might lower risk. But other studies have found that vitamin E supplements have no impact on cancer risk, and larger doses may increase risk for some kinds of heart disease. Some studies have also suggested that **selenium**, a mineral, might lower the risk of prostate cancer.

To study the possible effects of selenium and vitamin E on prostate cancer risk, doctors conducted the Selenium and Vitamin E Cancer Prevention Trial (SELECT). In this clinical trial, about 35,000 men were randomized to take one or both of these supplements or to take an inactive placebo. After an average of about 5 years of daily use, neither supplement was found to lower prostate cancer risk.

Taking any supplements can have risks and benefits. Before starting vitamins or other supplements, you should talk with your doctor.

Several studies are now looking at the possible effects of soy proteins (called **isoflavones**) on prostate cancer risk. The results of these studies are not yet available.

Medicines

Some drugs may also help reduce the risk of prostate cancer.

5 alpha-reductase inhibitors

5 alpha-reductase is the enzyme that changes testosterone into dihydrotestosterone (DHT). DHT is the hormone that causes the prostate to grow. 5 alpha-reductase inhibitors are drugs that block that enzyme and prevent the formation of DHT.

Finasteride (Proscar) is a 5 alpha-reductase inhibitor that is already used to treat benign prostatic hyperplasia (BPH). It is also available in a lower-dose form (called Propecia) to treat male pattern baldness.

The Prostate Cancer Prevention Trial (PCPT) was a large clinical trial designed to determine whether finasteride could lower the risk of prostate cancer. Half of the men in the study took finasteride each day for 7 years, and the other half took a placebo (sugar pill). At the end of the study, men taking finasteride were less likely to have prostate cancer than those getting the placebo. At first, it appeared that the men taking finasteride had slightly more cancers with high Gleason scores—cancers that looked like they were more likely to grow and spread. It is now believed that this is not true and men who took finasteride are not more likely to have a high-grade cancer develop. Researchers are still watching the men in the study to see if the men taking the drug lived longer. (Read more about the Gleason score in "How Is Prostate Cancer Diagnosed?" on pages 35–40.)

Finasteride was more likely to cause sexual **side effects** such as lowered sexual desire and impotence. But it seemed to help with urinary problems such as trouble urinating and leaking urine (incontinence).

Not all doctors agree that taking finasteride will help prevent prostate cancer. Men who are thinking about taking this drug should discuss it with their doctors. The results of the Prostate Cancer Prevention Trial will become clearer over the next few years.

Dutasteride (Avodart), another 5 alpha-reductase inhibitor, is currently being tested in a clinical trial to see if it can lower the risk of prostate cancer. Early results from this study reported this year indicate that it may have effects similar to that of finasteride.

Other drugs

In a small study, toremifene, an antiestrogen, decreased the risk of prostate cancer in men with high-grade prostatic intraepithelial neoplasia (PIN). A larger study to confirm this finding is ongoing. Other drugs that may help prevent prostate cancer are now being tested in clinical trials.

Can Prostate Cancer Be Found Early?

Screening refers to testing to find a disease such as cancer in people who do not have symptoms of that disease. For some types of cancer, screening can help find cancers in an early stage when they are more easily cured.

Prostate cancer can often be found early by testing the amount of **prostate-specific antigen (PSA)** in the blood. Another way to find prostate cancer is the **digital rectal examination (DRE),** in which your doctor puts a gloved finger into the rectum to feel the prostate gland. These 2 tests are described below in more detail. If the results of either one of these tests are abnormal, further testing is needed to determine whether cancer is present.

If prostate cancer is found during screening with the PSA test or DRE, your cancer will likely be at an early, more treatable stage than if no screening tests were done.

Since the use of **early detection** tests for prostate cancer became fairly common (about 1990), the prostate cancer death rate has dropped. But it isn't clear whether this drop is a direct result of screening or whether it is caused by something else, such as improvements in treatment.

There are limits to the prostate cancer screening tests used today. Neither the PSA test nor the DRE is 100% accurate. These tests can have abnormal results even when cancer is not present (known as **false positive** results). In addition, normal results can occur even when cancer is present (known as **false negative** results). Unclear test results can cause confusion and anxiety. False positive results can lead some men to undergo a prostate biopsy (with risks of pain, infection, and bleeding) when cancer is not present. And false negative results may give some men a false sense of security even though they actually have cancer.

The PSA test can definitely help spot many prostate cancers early; however, it cannot reveal how dangerous the cancer is. Finding and treating all prostate cancers early may seem like a no-brainer. But some prostate cancers grow so slowly that they would likely never cause problems. Because of an elevated PSA level, some men may receive a diagnosis of a prostate cancer that they would have never even known about at all. It would never have caused any symptoms or lead to their death. But they may still be treated with either surgery or radiation, either because the doctor can't be sure how aggressive (fast growing and fast spreading) the cancer might be, or because the men are uncomfortable not having any treatment.

Treatments like surgery and radiation can have side effects that seriously affect a man's quality of life. These treatments can lead to urinary, bowel, and/or sexual problems. In some men, these problems may be minimal and/or short-term, but for others these problems can be severe and long-lasting (or even permanent).

Doctors and patients are still struggling to decide who should receive treatment and who might be able to be followed without being treated right away (an approach called "watchful waiting" or "active surveillance"). Even when patients are not treated right away, they still need regular blood tests and prostate biopsies to determine the need for future treatment. These tests are linked with risks of anxiety, pain, infection, and bleeding.

Studies are under way to determine whether early detection tests for prostate cancer in large groups of men will lower the prostate cancer death rate. The most recent results from 2 large studies were conflicting and didn't offer clear answers.

Early results from a study conducted in the United States found that annual screening with PSA and DRE detected more prostate cancers, but it did not lower the death rate from prostate cancer. A European study did find a lower risk of death from prostate cancer with PSA screening (done about once every 4 years), but the researchers estimated that about 1,400 men would need to be screened (and 48 treated) in order to prevent one death from prostate cancer. Neither of these studies has shown that PSA screening helps men live longer (that it results in a lower overall death rate).

Prostate cancer tends to be a slow-growing cancer, so the effects of screening in these studies may become clearer in the coming years. Both of these studies are being continued to see if longer follow-up will give clearer results.

Recently, early results of a Swedish study of prostate cancer screening were published. One group of men was offered PSA testing every other year, with follow-up tests including biopsy if the PSA was over a certain level. This study did not test elderly men, that is, those older than 71 years of age were not tested. Cancer and death rates were compared between the group of men who were offered testing and the group that was not offered testing. After 15 years, the group offered testing had a lower risk of death from prostate cancer, but the overall death rate was the same for both groups.

At this time, the American Cancer Society (ACS) recommends that men thinking about prostate cancer screening should make informed decisions based on available information, discussion with their doctor, and their own views on the benefits and side effects of screening and treatment (see below).

Until more information is available, you and your doctor can decide whether you should have tests to screen for prostate cancer. There are many factors to take into account, including your age and health. If you are young and prostate cancer develops, it may shorten your life if it is not caught early. If you are older or in poor health, then prostate cancer may never become a major problem for you because it is often a slow-growing cancer.

American Cancer Society Recommendations for the Early Detection of Prostate Cancer

The American Cancer Society recommends that men have a chance to make an informed decision with their health care provider about whether to be screened for prostate cancer. The decision should be made after getting information about the uncertainties, risks, and potential benefits of prostate cancer screening. Men should not be screened unless they have received this information.

The discussion about screening should take place at age 50 for men who are at average risk for prostate cancer and are expected to live at least 10 more years.

This discussion should take place starting at age 45 for men at high risk for prostate cancer.

This group includes black men and men with a first-degree relative (father, brother, or son) who received a diagnosis of prostate cancer at an early age (younger than age 65).

This discussion should take place at age 40 for men at even higher risk (those with several first-degree relatives who had prostate cancer at an early age).

After this discussion, those men who want to be screened should be tested with the prostate-specific antigen (PSA) blood test. The digital rectal examination (DRE) may also be done as a part of screening.

If, after this discussion, a man is unable to decide whether testing is right for him, the screening decision can be made by the health care provider, who should take into account the patient's general health preferences and values.

Men who choose to be tested who have a PSA of less than 2.5 ng/mL, may only need to be retested every 2 years.

Screening should be done yearly for men whose PSA level is 2.5 ng/mL or higher.

Because prostate cancer grows slowly, those men without symptoms of prostate cancer who do not have a 10-year life expectancy should not be offered testing since they are not likely to benefit. Overall health status, and not age alone, is important when making decisions about screening.

Even after a decision about testing has been made, the discussion about the pros and cons of testing should be repeated as new information about the benefits and risks of testing becomes available. Further discussions are also needed to take into account changes in the patient's health, values, and preferences.

Prostate-Specific Antigen Blood Test

Prostate-specific antigen (PSA) is a substance made by cells in the prostate gland (it is made by normal cells and cancer cells). Although PSA is found mostly in semen, a small amount is also found in the blood. Most healthy men have levels under 4 ng/mL of blood. The chance of having prostate cancer goes up as the PSA level goes up.

When prostate cancer develops, the PSA level usually goes above 4. Still, a level below 4 does not mean that cancer isn't present—about 15% of men with a PSA below 4 will have prostate cancer on biopsy. Men with a PSA level in the borderline range between 4 and 10 have about a 1 in 4 chance of having prostate cancer. If the PSA is more than 10, the chance of having prostate cancer is greater than 50%.

The PSA level can also be increased by circumstances other than prostate cancer, such as the following:

Benign prostatic hyperplasia (BPH): BPH is a noncancerous enlargement of the prostate that many men get as they grow older.

Age: PSA levels will also normally go up slowly as men get older, even if they have no prostate abnormality.

Prostatitis: Prostatitis is an infection or inflammation of the prostate gland.

Ejaculation: Ejaculation can cause the PSA to go up for a short time, and then go down again. For this reason, some doctors will suggest that men abstain from ejaculation for 2 days before testing.

Some things cause PSA levels to go down (even when cancer is present), including the following:

- **Medicines:** Certain medicines used to treat BPH or urinary symptoms, such as finasteride (Proscar or Propecia) or dutasteride (Avodart). You should tell your doctor if you are taking these medicines, because they may lower PSA levels and require the doctor to adjust the reading.

- **Herbal mixtures:** Some herbal mixtures that are sold as dietary supplements "for prostate health" may also mask a high PSA level. This is why it is important to let your doctor know if you are taking any type of supplement. **Saw palmetto** (an herb used by some men to treat BPH) does not seem to interfere with the measurement of PSA.

- **Obesity:** Obese men tend to have lower PSA levels.

- **Aspirin:** Men taking aspirin regularly tend to have lower PSA levels. This effect is most pronounced in nonsmokers.

If your PSA level is high, your doctor may advise a prostate biopsy to find out if you have cancer (see the section, "How Is Prostate Cancer Diagnosed?"). Some doctors may consider using newer types of PSA tests (discussed on page 29) to help determine if you need a prostate biopsy, but not all doctors agree on how to use these other PSA tests. If your PSA test result is not normal, ask your doctor to assess (and discuss with you) your cancer risk and whether further tests are needed.

Percent-free PSA

PSA occurs in 2 major forms in the blood. One form is attached to blood proteins while the other circulates free (unattached). The **percent-free PSA (fPSA)** is the ratio of how much PSA circulates free compared with the total PSA level. The percentage of free PSA is lower in men who have prostate cancer than in those who do not have the disease.

If a man's PSA test results are in the borderline range (between 4 and 10), the fPSA is sometimes used to help decide whether a prostate biopsy is needed. A lower percent-free PSA means that the likelihood of having prostate cancer is higher and a biopsy is probably needed. Many doctors recommend biopsies for men whose percent-free PSA is 10% or less and advise that men consider a biopsy if it is between 10% and 25%. Using these cutoffs detects most cancers while helping some men to avoid unnecessary prostate biopsies. The percent-free PSA test is widely used, but not all doctors agree that 25% is the best cutoff point to decide on a biopsy.

A newer test, known as **complexed PSA**, measures the amount of PSA that is attached to other proteins.

PSA velocity

The **PSA velocity** is not a separate test. It is a measure of how fast the PSA rises over time. Even when the total PSA value isn't over 4, a high PSA velocity suggests that cancer may be present and a biopsy should be considered. For example, if your PSA was 1.7 on one test, and then a year later it was 3.8, this rapid rise may be cause for concern.

The PSA velocity can be useful if you are having the PSA test every year. For men whose initial PSA value is less than 4, a PSA velocity of 0.35 (ng/mL) per year or greater (for example, if values went from 2 to 2.4 to 2.8 over the course of 2 years) may be cause for concern. For men whose PSA value is between 4 and 10, a biopsy should be more strongly considered if it goes up faster than 0.75 (ng/mL) per year (for example, if values went from 4 to 4.8 to 5.6 over the course of 2 years). Most doctors believe that in order to get an accurate PSA velocity, the PSA levels should be measured on at least 3 occasions over a period of at least 18 months.

PSA density

PSA levels are higher in men with larger prostate glands. The **PSA density (PSAD)** is sometimes used for men with large prostate glands to try to adjust for this variable. The doctor measures the volume (size) of the prostate gland with transrectal ultrasound (discussed on page 33) and divides the PSA number by the prostate volume. A higher PSAD indicates a greater likelihood of cancer. PSAD has not been shown to be that useful. The percent-free PSA test has so far been shown to be more accurate.

Age-specific PSA ranges

PSA levels are normally higher in older men than in younger men, even when there is no cancer. A PSA result within the borderline range might be very worrisome in a 50-year-old man but cause less concern in an 80-year-old man. For this reason, some doctors have suggested comparing PSA results with results from other men of the same age.

The usefulness of age-specific PSA ranges is not well proven; therefore, most doctors and professional organizations (as well as the makers of the PSA tests) do not recommend their use at this time.

Using the PSA blood test after prostate cancer diagnosis

The PSA test is used mainly to detect prostate cancer early, but it is also useful in other situations:

In men with a diagnosis of prostate cancer, the PSA test can be used together with results of the clinical examination and tumor grade (from the biopsy) to help determine whether further tests (such as CT scans or bone scans) are needed.

- The PSA test can help determine whether your cancer is still confined to the prostate gland. If your PSA level is very high, your cancer has likely spread beyond the prostate. This information may affect your treatment options, since some forms of therapy (such as surgery and radiation) are not likely to be helpful if the cancer has spread to the lymph nodes, bones, or other organs.
- After surgery or radiation treatment, the PSA level can be watched to help determine

whether the treatment was successful. PSA levels normally fall to very low levels if the treatment removed or destroyed all of the prostate cancer cells. A rising PSA level (especially after surgery) likely means that prostate cancer cells are present and your cancer has come back.

- If you choose an "active surveillance" approach to treatment, the PSA level can be used to help decide whether the cancer is growing and if active treatment should be considered.

- During hormone therapy or chemotherapy, the PSA level can help indicate how well the treatment is working or when it may be time to try a different form of treatment.

If prostate cancer has recurred after treatment, or if it has spread outside of the prostate (metastatic disease), the actual PSA number is probably not as important as whether it changes. The PSA number does not predict whether a person will have symptoms or how long he will live. Many people have very high PSA values and feel just fine. Other people have low values and have symptoms. With advanced disease, it may be more important to examine how the PSA level is changing rather than the actual number.

Digital Rectal Examination

For a digital rectal examination (DRE), a doctor inserts a gloved, lubricated finger into the rectum to feel for any bumps or hard areas on the prostate that might be cancer. The prostate gland is found just in front of the rectum, and most cancers begin in the back part of the gland, which can be felt during a rectal exam. This examination is uncomfortable, but it is not painful and takes only a short time.

DRE is less effective than the PSA blood test in finding prostate cancer, but it can sometimes find cancers in men with normal PSA levels. For this reason, it may be included as a part of prostate cancer screening.

The DRE can also be used once a man is known to have prostate cancer to try to determine whether it has spread to nearby tissues and to detect cancer that has come back after treatment.

Transrectal Ultrasound

Transrectal ultrasound (TRUS) uses sound waves to make an image of the prostate on a video screen. For this test, a small probe that gives off sound waves is placed in the rectum. The sound waves enter the prostate and create echoes that are picked up by the probe. A computer turns the pattern of echoes into a black and white image of the prostate.

The procedure takes only a few minutes and is done in a doctor's office or outpatient clinic. You will feel some pressure when the TRUS probe is placed in your rectum, but it is usually not painful.

TRUS is not used as a screening test for prostate cancer because it doesn't often show early cancer. Instead, it is most commonly used during a prostate biopsy (described in the next section). TRUS is used to guide the biopsy needles into the right area of the prostate.

TRUS is useful in other situations as well. It can be used to measure the size of the prostate gland, which can help determine the PSA density and may also affect a man's treatment options. It is also used as a guide during some forms of treatment such as cryosurgery.

Diagnosis and Staging

How Is Prostate Cancer Diagnosed?

Signs and Symptoms of Prostate Cancer

Early prostate cancer usually causes no **symptoms** and is most often found by a prostate-specific antigen (PSA) test and/or digital rectal examination (DRE). Some advanced prostate cancers can slow or weaken the urinary stream or make you need to urinate more often. But these symptoms are more frequently caused by noncancerous diseases of the prostate, such as benign prostatic hyperplasia (BPH).

If the prostate cancer is advanced, you might have **hematuria** (blood in your urine) or **impotence** (trouble getting an erection). Advanced prostate cancer commonly spreads to the bones, which can cause pain in the hips, back (spine), chest (ribs), or other areas. Cancer that has spread to the spine can also press on the spinal nerves, which can result in weakness or numbness in the legs or feet, or even loss of bladder or bowel control.

Other diseases can also cause many of these same symptoms. It is important to tell your doctor if you have any of these problems so that the cause can be found and treated.

If certain symptoms or the results of early detection tests—the PSA blood test and/or DRE—suggest that you might have prostate cancer, your doctor will do a prostate biopsy to determine whether the disease is present.

The Prostate Biopsy

A biopsy is a procedure in which a sample of body tissue is removed and then examined under a microscope. A core needle biopsy is the main method used to diagnose prostate cancer. It is usually done by a urologist, a surgeon who treats cancers of the genital and urinary tract, which includes the prostate gland. Using transrectal ultrasound (described in the section on early detection of prostate cancer, page 33) to "see" the prostate gland, the doctor quickly inserts a needle through the wall of the rectum into the prostate gland. When the needle is pulled out, it removes a small cylinder of tissue, usually about $1/2$-inch long and $1/16$-inch across. This process is repeated from 8 to 18 times, although most urologists will take about 12 samples. These samples are sent to the laboratory to determine whether cancer is present.

Though the procedure sounds painful, it may only cause a very brief, uncomfortable sensation because it is done with a special spring-loaded biopsy instrument. The device inserts and removes the needles in a fraction of a second. Most doctors who do the biopsy will numb the area first by injecting a local anesthetic alongside the prostate.

You might want to ask your doctor if he or she plans to use an anesthetic during the procedure.

Some doctors will perform the biopsy through the **perineum**, the skin between the rectum and the **scrotum**. The doctor will place his or her finger in your rectum to feel the prostate and then insert the biopsy needle through a small **incision** (cut) in the skin of the perineum. The doctor will also use a local **anesthetic** to numb the area.

The biopsy itself takes about 15 minutes and is usually done in the doctor's office. You will likely be given antibiotics to take before the biopsy and for a day or 2 after to reduce the risk of infection.

For a few days after the procedure, you may feel some soreness in the area and will likely notice blood in your urine. You may also have some light bleeding from your rectum. Many men also see some blood in their **semen** or have rust-colored semen, which can last for several weeks after the biopsy.

Your biopsy samples will be sent to a pathology laboratory. There, a pathologist (a doctor who specializes in diagnosing disease in tissue samples) will determine whether there are cancer cells in your biopsy by looking at the samples under the microscope. If cancer is present, the pathologist will also assign it a grade (see more about cancer grades on pages 38–39). Getting the results usually takes at least 1 to 3 days, but it can take longer.

Even with many samples, biopsies can still sometimes miss a cancer if none of the biopsy needles pass through it. This is known as a false negative result. If your doctor still strongly suspects prostate cancer (owing to a very high PSA level, for example), a repeat biopsy may be needed.

Grading the prostate cancer

Almost all pathologists grade prostate cancers according to the **Gleason system**. This system assigns a **Gleason grade**, using numbers from 1 to 5 based on how much the cells in the cancerous tissue look like normal prostate tissue.

- If the cancerous tissue looks much like normal prostate tissue, a grade of 1 is assigned.
- If the cancer lacks these normal features and its cells seem to be spread haphazardly through the prostate, it is called a grade 5 tumor.
- Grades 2 through 4 have features in between these extremes.

Because prostate cancers often have areas with different grades, a **grade** is assigned to the 2 areas that make up most of the cancer. These 2 grades are added together to yield the **Gleason score** (also called the Gleason sum), which will be between 2 and 10. There are some exceptions to this rule. If the highest grade takes up most (95% or higher) of the biopsy, the grade for that area is counted twice in the Gleason score. Also, if 3 grades are present in a biopsy core, the highest grade is always included in the Gleason score, even if most of the core is taken up by areas of cancer with lower grades.

- Cancers with Gleason scores of 2 to 4 are sometimes called well-differentiated or *low-*

grade. Cancers with Gleason scores of 2 to 4 are rarely diagnosed in needle biopsies.

- Cancers with Gleason scores of 5 to 7 may be called moderately differentiated or *intermediate-grade.*
- Cancers with Gleason scores of 8 to 10 may be called poorly differentiated or **high-grade**.

The higher your Gleason score, the more likely it is that your cancer will grow and spread quickly.

Other elements of a biopsy report

The pathologist's report contains the grade of the cancer (if it is present) but it also often contains other pieces of information that may give a better idea of the scope of the cancer. This information can include the following:

- the number of biopsy core samples that contain cancer (for example, "7 of 12")
- the percentage of cancer in each of the cores
- whether the cancer is on one side (left or right) of the prostate or both sides (bilateral)

Suspicious results

Sometimes when the pathologist looks at the prostate cells under the microscope, they don't look cancerous, but they're not quite normal, either. These results are often reported as suspicious. They generally fall into 2 categories: prostatic intraepithelial neoplasia (PIN) or atypical small acinar proliferation (ASAP).

In PIN, there are changes in how the prostate cells look under the microscope, but the abnormal cells don't look like they've grown into other parts of the prostate (like cancer cells would). PIN is often divided into low-grade and high-grade. Many men begin to have low-grade PIN develop at an early age but do not necessarily develop prostate cancer. The importance of low-grade PIN in relation to prostate cancer is still unclear.

If high-grade PIN is found on a biopsy, there is about a 20% to 30% chance that cancer may already be present somewhere else in the prostate gland. This is why doctors often carefully observe men with high-grade PIN and may advise a repeat prostate biopsy, especially if samples were not taken from all parts of the prostate during the original biopsy.

Atypical small acinar proliferation (ASAP)—another finding sometimes reported on a prostate biopsy—is sometimes just called atypia. In ASAP, the cells look like they might be cancerous when viewed under the microscope, but there are too few of them to be sure. If ASAP is found, there's about a 40% to 50% chance that cancer is also present in the prostate, which is why many doctors recommend getting a repeat biopsy within a few months.

How Is Prostate Cancer Staged?

The **stage** (extent) of a cancer is one of the most important factors in choosing treatment options and predicting a patient's outlook. If your prostate biopsy confirms that you have cancer, more tests may be done to find out how far it has spread within the prostate, to nearby tissues, or to other parts of the body. This process is called **staging**.

Your doctor will use the results of your DRE, PSA level, and Gleason score to determine the likelihood that your cancer has spread outside of the prostate. This information is used to decide which other tests (if any) need to be done before deciding on a treatment. Men with a normal DRE result, a low PSA, and a low Gleason score may not need any other tests because the chance that the cancer has spread is so low.

Medical History and Physical Examination

The physical examination, especially the digital rectal examination (DRE), is an important part of prostate cancer staging. By performing a DRE, your doctor can sometimes tell whether the cancer is only on one side of the prostate, whether it is present on both sides, or whether it is likely to have spread beyond the prostate gland to nearby tissues. The DRE is always used together with the PSA blood test for early detection of prostate cancer and is discussed on pages 32–33. Your doctor may also examine other areas of your body to see whether the cancer has spread.

Your doctor will also ask you about symptoms such as urinary problems or bone pain, which could suggest the possibility that the cancer has spread to your bones.

Imaging Tests Used for Prostate Cancer Staging

Not all men with prostate cancer need to have **imaging tests**, but for those who do, the following tests are sometimes used.

Radionuclide bone scan

When prostate cancer spreads to distant sites, it often goes to the bones first. (Even when prostate cancer spreads to the bone, it is still called prostate cancer, not bone cancer.) A radionuclide bone scan can help show whether cancer has reached the bones.

When a radionuclide **bone scan** is performed, a small amount of low-level radioactive material is injected into a vein (intravenously, or IV). The substance settles in damaged bone tissue throughout the entire skeleton over the course of a couple of hours. The patient then lies on a table for about 30 minutes while a special camera detects the radioactivity and creates a picture of his skeleton.

Areas of bone damage will appear as "hot spots" on the skeleton—that is, they attract the radioactivity. Hot spots may also suggest the presence of metastatic cancer, but arthritis or other bone diseases can cause the same pattern. To tell the difference between these conditions, the **cancer care team** may use other imaging tests such as simple **x-rays** or computed tomography (CT) or magnetic resonance imaging (MRI) scans to get a better look at the areas that light up, or they may even take biopsy samples of the bone.

The injection is the only uncomfortable part of the scanning procedure. The radioactive material is passed out of the body in the urine over the next few days. The amount of radioactivity used is very low, so it carries very little risk to the patient or to others. But you still may want to ask your doctor if you should take any special precautions after having this test.

Computed tomography

The **computed tomography (CT** or **CAT scan)** is a special kind of x-ray that gives detailed, cross-sectional images of your body. Instead of taking one picture, like a standard x-ray, a CT scanner takes many pictures of the part of your body being studied as it rotates around you. A computer then combines these pictures into images of slices of the part of your body being studied.

Before the first set of pictures is taken, you may be asked to drink 1 or 2 pints of **contrast solution**. This solution helps outline the intestine so that it looks different from any tumors. You may also receive an **intravenous (IV) line** through which a different kind of contrast material is injected. This material helps better outline structures in your body. You will also need to drink enough liquid to have a full bladder. A full bladder will keep the bowel away from the area of the prostate gland.

The IV contrast can cause your body to feel flushed (a feeling of warmth with some redness of the skin). A few people are allergic and get hives. Rarely, more serious reactions, like trouble breathing or low blood pressure, can occur. Medication can be given to prevent and treat allergic reactions, so be sure to tell your doctor if you have ever had a reaction to any contrast material used for x-rays. It is also important to let your doctor know about any other allergies.

CT scans take longer than regular x-rays. You need to lie still on a table while they are being done. During the test, the table moves in and out of the scanner, a ring-shaped machine that completely surrounds the table. You might feel a bit confined by the ring you have to lie in while the pictures are being taken.

CT scanning can help reveal whether prostate cancer has spread into nearby **lymph nodes**. If there is a **recurrence** of cancer after your treatment, the CT scan may help determine whether it is growing into other organs or structures in your **pelvis**. On the other hand, CT scans rarely provide useful information about newly diagnosed prostate cancers that are likely to be confined to the prostate based on other findings (DRE result, PSA level, and Gleason score). CT scans are not as useful as MRI for looking at the prostate gland itself.

Magnetic resonance imaging

Magnetic resonance imaging (MRI) uses radio waves and strong magnets instead of x-rays. The energy from the radio waves is absorbed by the body and then released in a pattern formed by the type of body tissue and by certain diseases. A computer translates the pattern into a very detailed image of parts of the body. This produces cross-sectional slices of the body like a CT scanner, but it can also show slices (views) from several angles. Like a CT scan, a contrast material might be injected, but this step is done less often.

MRI scans can be very helpful in looking at prostate cancer. They can produce a very clear picture of the prostate and show whether the cancer has spread outside the prostate into the seminal vesicles or the bladder. This information can be very important for your doctors in planning your treatment. But like CT scans, MRI scans may not provide useful information about newly diagnosed prostate cancers that are likely to be localized (confined to the prostate) based on other factors.

MRI scans take longer than CT scans—often up to an hour. During the scan, you need to lie still inside a narrow tube, which is confining and can be upsetting for people who don't like enclosed spaces. The machine also makes clicking and buzzing noises. Some places provide headphones with music to block out this noise. To improve the accuracy of the MRI, many doctors will place a probe, called an endorectal coil, inside the rectum. This probe must stay in place for 30 to 45 minutes and can be uncomfortable.

ProstaScint™ scan

Like the bone scan, the **ProstaScint scan** uses an injection of low-level radioactive material to find cancer that has spread beyond the prostate. Both tests look for areas of the body where the radioactive material collects, but they work in different ways.

While the radioactive material used for the bone scan is attracted to bone, the material for the ProstaScint scan is attracted to prostate cells in the body. It is attached to a **monoclonal antibody**, a type of man-made protein that recognizes and sticks to a particular substance. In this case, the antibody sticks to **prostate-specific membrane antigen (PSMA)**, a substance found at high levels in both normal and cancerous prostate cells.

After the material is injected, the patient will be asked to lie on a table while a special camera creates an image of the body. This scan is usually done about half an hour after the injection and again 3 to 5 days later.

The advantage of this test is that it can find prostate cancer cells in lymph nodes and other soft (non-bone) organs. Because the antibody sticks only to prostate cancer cells, other cancers or benign problems should not cause abnormal results. But the test is not always accurate, and the results can sometimes be confusing.

Most doctors do not recommend the ProstaScint scan for men who have just received a diagnosis of prostate cancer. But it may be useful after treatment if the blood PSA level begins to rise and other tests are not able to find the exact location of your cancer. Doctors may not order this test if they believe it will not be helpful for a given patient.

Lymph Node Biopsy

In a lymph node biopsy, one or more lymph nodes are removed to see if they contain cancer cells. This procedure, also called a lymph node dissection or

lymphadenectomy, is sometimes done to determine whether the cancer has spread from the prostate to nearby lymph nodes. If cancer cells are found in a lymph node, surgery is not likely to cure the cancer, so other treatment options are considered. Lymph node biopsies are rarely done unless your doctor is concerned that the cancer has spread. There are several ways to biopsy lymph nodes.

Surgical biopsy

The surgeon may remove lymph nodes through an incision in the lower part of your abdomen. This procedure is often done in the same operation as the radical prostatectomy. (See the section, "How Is Prostate Cancer Treated?" for information about radical prostatectomy.)

If the surgeon has a reason to suspect that the cancer may have spread (such as a PSA level over 20 or a Gleason score over 7), he or she may remove some lymph nodes before attempting to remove the prostate gland. A pathologist will examine the nodes while the patient is still under **anesthesia** to help the surgeon decide whether to continue with the radical prostatectomy. This technique is called a **frozen section** examination because the tissue sample is frozen before thin slices are taken to check under a microscope. If the nodes contain cancer, the operation is usually stopped (and the prostate is left in place). This choice is often made because removing the prostate would be unlikely to cure the cancer, and it could still result in serious complications or side effects.

If the PSA is less than 20 and the Gleason score isn't high, the chance that the cancer has already spread is low. In that case, surgeons do not often request a frozen section examination and instead send the lymph nodes to the laboratory to be examined along with the removed prostate gland. The test results are usually available 3 to 7 days after surgery.

Laparoscopic biopsy

A **laparoscope** is a long, slender tube with a small video camera on the end that is inserted into the abdomen to allow the surgeon to see inside without making a large incision. Other small incisions are made to insert long instruments to remove the lymph nodes. The surgeon removes all of the lymph nodes around the prostate gland and sends them to the pathologist. Because there are no large incisions, most people recover fully in only 1 or 2 days, and the operation leaves very small scars. A laparoscopic biopsy is not common, but it is sometimes used when it's important to know the lymph node status and radical prostatectomy is not planned (such as for certain men who choose treatment with radiation therapy).

Fine needle aspiration

If your lymph nodes appear enlarged on an imaging test (CT or MRI), a specially trained radiologist may take a sample of cells from an enlarged lymph node by using a technique called **fine needle aspiration (FNA)**. To do this, the doctor uses the CT scan image to guide a long, thin needle through the skin in the lower abdomen and into an enlarged lymph node. A syringe attached to the needle allows the doctor to take a small tissue sample from the node. Before the needle is placed, your skin will be numbed with local anesthesia. You will be able to return home a few hours after the procedure. This method is not used very often.

The AJCC TNM Staging System

A staging system is a standard way in which the cancer care team describes the extent to which a cancer has spread. While there are several different staging systems for prostate cancer, the most widely used system is the American Joint Committee on Cancer (AJCC) TNM System.

The TNM System describes 3 key pieces of information:

- **T** refers to the size of the **tumor**.
- **N** describes how far the cancer has spread to nearby **lymph nodes** (N category). Lymph nodes are small, bean-shaped collections of immune system cells that are important to fighting infections.
- **M** indicates whether the cancer has spread (**metastasized**) to other organs of the body.

The overall stage takes all 3 categories into account, along with the Gleason score and the PSA level (described in the section, "How Is Prostate Cancer Diagnosed?").

There are actually 2 types of staging for prostate cancer. The **clinical stage** is your doctor's best estimate of the extent of your disease, based on the results of the physical examination (including DRE), laboratory tests, prostate biopsy, and any imaging tests you have had.

If you have surgery, your doctors can also determine the **pathologic stage**, which is based on the surgery and examination of the removed tissue. This means that if you have surgery, the stage of your cancer might actually change afterward (if cancer was found in a place it wasn't suspected, for example). Pathologic staging is likely to be more accurate than clinical staging, as it allows your doctor to get a firsthand impression of the extent of your disease. This is one possible advantage of having surgery (radical prostatectomy) as opposed to radiation therapy or watchful waiting (expectant management).

Both types of staging use the same categories (but the T1 category is not used in pathologic staging).

T categories

There are 4 categories for describing the local extent of the prostate tumor, ranging from T1 to T4. Most of these categories have subcategories as well.

> **T1:** Your doctor can't feel the tumor or see it with imaging such as transrectal ultrasound.
>> **T1a:** The cancer is found incidentally (by accident) during a transurethral resection of the prostate (often abbreviated as TURP) that was done for benign prostatic hyperplasia (BPH).

Cancer is present in less than 5% of the tissue removed.

T1b: The cancer is found during a TURP but is present in more than 5% of the tissue removed.

T1c: The cancer is found by needle biopsy that was done because of an increased PSA.

T2: Your doctor can feel the cancer when a digital rectal examination (DRE) is done, but it still appears to be confined to the prostate gland.

T2a: The cancer is in one half or less of only one side (left or right) of your prostate.

T2b: The cancer is in more than half of only one side (left or right) of your prostate.

T2c: The cancer is in both sides of your prostate.

T3: The cancer has begun to grow and spread outside your prostate and may involve the seminal vesicles.

T3a: The cancer extends outside the prostate but not to the seminal vesicles.

T3b: The cancer has spread to the seminal vesicles.

T4: The cancer has grown into tissues next to your prostate (other than the seminal vesicles), such as the bladder sphincter (muscle that helps control urination), the rectum, and/or the wall of the pelvis.

N categories

N0: The cancer has not spread to any lymph nodes.

N1: The cancer has spread to one or more regional (nearby) lymph nodes in the pelvis.

M categories

M0: The cancer has not spread beyond the regional lymph nodes.

M1: The cancer has spread beyond the regional nodes.

M1a: The cancer has spread to distant (outside of the pelvis) lymph nodes.

M1b: The cancer has spread to the bones.

M1c: The cancer has spread to other organs such as lungs, liver, or brain (with or without spread to the bones).

Stage Grouping

Once the T, N, and M categories have been determined, this information is combined, along with the Gleason score and PSA, in a process called stage grouping. If the Gleason score or PSA results are not available, the stage can be based on the T, N, and M categories. The overall stage is expressed in Roman numerals from I (the least advanced) to IV (the most advanced). This process is done to help determine treatment options and the outlook for survival or cure.

Stage I

One of the following applies:

T1, N0, M0, Gleason score 6 or less, PSA less than 10: The doctor can't feel the tumor or see it with imaging such as transrectal ultrasound (it was either found during a transurethral resection or was diagnosed by needle biopsy done for a high PSA test result) [T1]. The cancer is still within the prostate and has not spread to lymph nodes [N0] or elsewhere in the body [M0]. The Gleason score is 6 or less and the PSA level is less than 10.

OR

T2a, N0, M0, Gleason score 6 or less, PSA less than 10: The tumor can be felt on DRE or seen on transrectal ultrasound and is in one half or less of only one side (left or right) of your prostate [T2a]. The cancer is still within the prostate and has not spread to lymph nodes [N0] or elsewhere in the body [M0]. The Gleason score is 6 or less and the PSA level is less than 10.

Stage IIA

One of the following applies:

T1, N0, M0, Gleason score of 7, PSA less than 20: The doctor can't feel the tumor or see it with imaging such as transrectal ultrasound (it was either found during a transurethral resection or was diagnosed by needle biopsy done for a high PSA level) [T1]. The cancer has not spread to nearby lymph nodes [N0] or elsewhere in the body [M0].The tumor has a Gleason score of 7. The PSA level is less than 20.

OR

T1, N0, M0, Gleason score of 6 or less, PSA at least 10 but less than 20: The doctor can't feel the tumor or see it with imaging such as transrectal ultrasound (it was either found during a transurethral resection or was diagnosed by needle biopsy done for a high PSA test result) [T1]. The cancer has not spread to nearby lymph nodes [N0] or elsewhere in the body [M0]. The tumor has a Gleason score of 6 or less. The PSA level is at least 10 but less than 20.

OR

T2a or T2b, N0, M0, Gleason score of 7 or less, PSA less than 20: The tumor can be felt on DRE or seen on transrectal ultrasound and is in only one side of the prostate [T2a or T2b]. The cancer has not spread to nearby lymph nodes [N0] or elsewhere in the body [M0]. It has a Gleason score of 7 or less. The PSA level is less than 20.

Stage IIB

One of the following applies:

T2c, N0, M0, any Gleason score, any PSA: The tumor can be felt on DRE or seen on transrectal ultrasound and is in both sides of the prostate [T2c]. The cancer has not spread to nearby lymph nodes [N0] or elsewhere in the body [M0]. The tumor can have any Gleason score and the PSA can be any value.

OR

T1 or T2, N0, M0, any Gleason score, PSA of 20 or more: The cancer has not yet begun to spread outside the prostate. It may (or may not) be felt by DRE or seen on transrectal ultrasound [T1 or T2] The cancer has not spread to nearby lymph nodes [N0] or elsewhere in the body [M0]. The tumor can have any Gleason score. The PSA level is at least 20.

OR

T1 or T2, N0, M0, Gleason score of 8 or higher, any PSA: The cancer has not yet begun to spread outside the prostate. It may (or may not) be felt by digital rectal examination or seen on transrectal ultrasound [T1 or T2]. The cancer has not spread to nearby lymph nodes [N0] or elsewhere in the body [M0]. The Gleason score is 8 or higher. The PSA can be any value.

Stage III

T3, N0, M0, any Gleason score, any PSA: The cancer has begun to spread outside the prostate and may have spread to the seminal vesicles [T3], but it has not spread to the lymph nodes [N0] or elsewhere in the body [M0]. The tumor can have any Gleason score and the PSA can be any value.

Stage IV

One of the following applies:

T4, N0, M0, any Gleason score, any PSA:
The cancer has spread to tissues next to the prostate (other than the seminal vesicles), such as the bladder's external sphincter (muscle that helps control urination), rectum, and/or the wall of the pelvis [T4]. The cancer has not spread to nearby lymph nodes [N0] or elsewhere in the body [M0]. The tumor can have any Gleason score and the PSA can be any value.

OR

Any T, N1, M0, any Gleason score, any PSA: The tumor may be growing into tissues near the prostate [any T]. The cancer has spread to the lymph nodes (N1) but has not spread elsewhere in the body [M0]. The tumor can have any Gleason score and the PSA can be any value.

OR

Any T, any N, M1, any Gleason score, any PSA: The cancer may be growing into tissues near the prostate [any T] and may have spread to nearby lymph nodes [any N]. It has spread to other, more distant sites in the body [M1]. The tumor can have any Gleason score and the PSA can be any value.

Other staging systems

In addition to the TNM system, other systems have been used to stage prostate cancer. The **Whitmore-Jewett staging system**, which stages prostate cancer as A, B, C, or D, was commonly used in the past, but most prostate specialists now use the TNM system. If your doctors use the Whitmore-Jewett system, ask them to translate it into the TNM system or to explain how their staging will determine your treatment options.

Five-Year Relative Survival Rates by Stage

The National Cancer Institute (NCI) maintains a large national database on survival statistics for different types of cancer. This database does not group cancers by AJCC stage, but instead groups cancers into local, regional and distant stages.

Local stage means that there is no sign that the cancer has spread outside of the prostate. This corresponds to AJCC stages I and II. Almost 9 out of 10 prostate cancers are found in this early stage. If the cancer has spread from the prostate to nearby areas, it is called **regional stage**. This includes stage III and the stage IV cancers that haven't spread to distant parts of the body, such as T4 tumors and cancers that have spread to nearby lymph nodes (N1). **Distant stage** includes the rest of the stage IV cancers—all cancers that have spread to distant lymph nodes, bone, or other organs (M1).

Five-Year Relative Survival Rates
According to Stage at Time of Diagnosis

Local	100%
Regional	100%
Distant	31%

The 5-year survival rate refers to the percentage of patients who live at least 5 years after their cancer is diagnosed. These rates are used to create a standard way of discussing prognosis (outlook). Of course, many of these patients live much longer than 5 years after diagnosis. Five-year relative survival rates compare the observed survival with that expected for people without the cancer. That means that relative survival only talks about deaths from the cancer in question. This is a more accurate way to describe the outlook for patients with a certain cancer.

Five-year survival rates are based on cancers diagnosed and first treated more than 5 years ago. Improvements in treatment since then may result in a better outlook for patients with recently diagnosed cancers.

Treatment

How Is Prostate Cancer Treated?

Making Treatment Decisions

Once your prostate cancer has been diagnosed, graded, and staged, you have a lot to think about before you and your doctor choose a treatment plan. You may feel that you must make a decision quickly, but it is important to give yourself time to absorb the information you have just learned. Ask questions of your cancer care team. Read the section, "What Should You Ask Your Doctor About Prostate Cancer?" on page 135.

The treatment you choose for prostate cancer should take into account the following factors:
- your age and expected life span
- any other serious health conditions you may have
- the stage and grade of your cancer
- your feelings (and your doctor's opinion) about the need to treat the cancer
- the likelihood that each type of treatment will cure your cancer (or provide some other measure of benefit)
- your feelings about the side effects common with each treatment

You may want to get a second opinion about the best treatment option for your situation, especially if there are several choices available to you. Prostate cancer is a complex disease, and doctors may differ in their opinions regarding the best treatment options. Speaking with doctors who specialize in different kinds of treatment may be helpful. You will want to weigh the benefits of each treatment against its possible outcomes, side effects, and risks.

Expectant Management (Watchful Waiting) and Active Surveillance

Because prostate cancer often grows very slowly, some men (especially those who are older or have other serious health problems) may never need treatment for their prostate cancer. Instead, their doctors may recommend approaches known as **expectant management**, **watchful waiting**, or **active surveillance**. Until recently, watchful waiting usually meant waiting until the cancer was causing symptoms before starting any treatment. Now, it is more common to watch the patient closely with regular PSA tests, digital rectal exams, and ultra-sounds to see if the cancer is growing. If the cancer does seem to be growing or getting worse, treatment may be recommended. Some doctors still consider this approach to be watchful waiting, while others consider this approach different from watchful waiting and call it "active surveillance." Not every doctor means the same thing when using the term "watchful waiting," so it is important to ask your doctor what he or she means by this term. Either of these approaches may be recommended if your cancer is not causing any symptoms, is expected to grow very slowly, and is small and contained within one area of the prostate.

Neither of these approaches is likely to be a good option if you are young, healthy, and/or have a fast-growing cancer (for example, a high Gleason score).

At this time, active surveillance is a reasonable option for some men with slow-growing cancers because it is not known whether treating the cancer with surgery or radiation will actually help them live longer. These treatments have definite risks and side effects that may outweigh the possible benefits for some men. Some men are not comfortable with this approach and are willing to accept the possible side effects of active treatments in order to try to remove or destroy the cancer.

With active surveillance, your cancer will be carefully monitored. Usually, this approach includes a doctor visit with a prostate-specific antigen (PSA) blood test and digital rectal examination (DRE) about every 3 to 6 months. Transrectal ultrasound–guided prostate biopsies may be done every year as well. Treatment is started if the cancer seems to be growing or getting worse, based on either a rising PSA, a change in the rectal exam, or biopsy results. On biopsies, an increase in the Gleason score or extent of tumor (based on the number of biopsies containing tumor) are both signals to start treatment. This treatment usually involves surgery or radiation therapy. Active surveillance allows the patient to be observed for a time, only treating those men who have a serious form of the cancer. This approach allows men with a less serious cancer avoid the side effects of treatment that may not have helped them live longer. A possible downside of this approach is that there's a chance it could allow the cancer to become more advanced. This choice could limit your treatment options such as surgery.

Right now, not all experts agree how often testing should occur for active surveillance. There is also debate about when is the best time to start therapy. Still, several early studies have shown that men who choose active surveillance and go on to be treated do just as well as those who decide to start treatment right away. In the near future, we hope to have a better idea of the pros and cons of active surveillance versus active treatment. A large study sponsored by the National Cancer Institute and the Veterans Affairs Cooperative Studies Program is now looking into how active treatment affects survival and quality of life of prostate cancer patients of different ages. The Prostatic Intervention Versus Observation Trial (PIVOT) is still in progress. Studies are under way to determine the best approach for monitoring patients on active surveillance, and this research should shed more light on the issue.

Surgery

Radical **prostatectomy** is designed to cure prostate cancer. This operation is used most often if the cancer is not believed to have spread outside of the gland (stage T1 or T2 cancers). The procedure includes removal of the entire prostate gland plus some of the tissue around it, including the seminal vesicles.

Radical retropubic prostatectomy

Radical retropubic prostatectomy is the operation used by most urologic surgeons (urologists). During the operation, the patient is either under general anesthesia (asleep) or is given spinal or epidural anesthesia (numbing the lower half of the body), along with sedation during the surgery.

For a radical retropubic prostatectomy, the surgeon makes a skin incision in the lower abdomen, from the belly button down to the pubic bone. If there is a reasonable chance the cancer may have spread to the lymph nodes (based on the PSA level, DRE, and biopsy results), the surgeon may remove lymph nodes from around the prostate at this time. If any of the nodes contain cancer cells, which means the cancer has spread, the surgeon may elect not to continue with the surgery, because it is unlikely that the cancer can be cured.

The surgeon will pay close attention to the 2 tiny bundles of nerves that run on either side of the prostate. These nerves control erections. If a patient is able to have erections before surgery, the surgeon will try not to injure these nerves (known as a "nerve-sparing" approach). If the cancer is growing into or very close to the nerves the surgeon will need to remove them. If they are both removed, the patient will be impotent (unable to have a spontaneous erection). This means that he

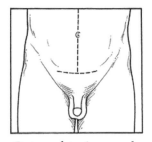 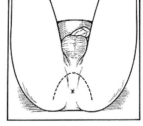

Retropubic Approach   Perineal Approach

will need help (such as medications or pumps) to have erections. If the nerves on one side are removed, there is still a chance of keeping the ability to have an erection. If neither nerve bundle is removed, the patient may be able to function normally. Usually it takes at least a few months to a year after surgery to have an erection because the nerves have been handled during the operation and won't work properly for a while.

Radical perineal prostatectomy

With radical perineal prostatectomy, the surgeon makes an incision in the skin between the anus and scrotum (the perineum), as shown in the picture above. This approach is used less often because the nerves cannot easily be spared and lymph nodes cannot be removed. But it is often a shorter operation and might be an option if the patient does not want the nerve-sparing procedure and lymph node removal is not required. It also might be used if a patient has other medical conditions that make retropubic surgery difficult. If done correctly, it can be just as curative as the **retropubic approach**.

Radical retropubic and perineal prostatectomy procedures usually take from 1½ to 4 hours. The perineal operation usually takes less time than the retropubic operation, and may result in less pain afterward. After surgery, a hospital stay of about 3 days is required, and the patient will probably be away from work for about 3 to 5 weeks.

In most cases, patients are able to donate their own blood before surgery. This blood can be returned to the patient during an operation, if it is needed.

After the surgery, while the patient is still under anesthesia, a **catheter** is placed in the penis to help drain the bladder. The catheter usually stays in place for 1 to 2 weeks while healing takes place. The patient can urinate on his own after the catheter is removed.

Laparoscopic radical prostatectomy

Both the radical retropubic prostatectomy and the radical perineal prostatectomy use an "open" technique, in which the surgeon makes a long incision to remove the prostate. Another technique, known as **laparoscopic radical prostatectomy (LRP)**, uses several smaller incisions, through which special long instruments are inserted to remove the prostate. One of the instruments has a small video camera on the end, which allows the surgeon to see inside the abdomen.

Laparoscopic prostatectomy has some advantages over the usual open radical prostatectomy, including less blood loss and pain, shorter hospital stays (usually no more than a day), and faster recovery times (although the catheter will be needed for about the same amount of time). LRP offers very good lighting and magnification, which can help the surgeon better decide which areas need to be removed.

Still, LRP is a challenging operation for surgeons to learn and usually requires a bit more time for the patient to be on the operating table (and under anesthesia). Another possible drawback is that it does not allow the surgeon to use the sense of touch while operating or to have the same freedom of motion with his or her hands.

LRP has been used in the United States since 1999 and is more frequently being done both in community and university centers. In experienced hands, LRP appears to be as good as open radical prostatectomy, although long-term results from procedures done in the United States are not currently available. Early studies report that the rates of side effects from LRP seem to be about the same as those associated with open prostatectomy. Recovery of bladder control may be slightly delayed with this approach. A nerve-sparing approach is possible with LRP, increasing the chance of normal erections after the operation.

Robotic-assisted laparoscopic radical prostatectomy

An even newer approach is to perform LRP remotely by using a robotic interface (called the da Vinci system). The surgeon sits at a panel near the operating table and controls robotic arms to perform the operation through several small incisions in the patient's abdomen. For the patient, there is little difference between direct and remote (robotic) LRP, either during surgery or recovery.

For the surgeon, the robotic system may provide more maneuverability and more precision when moving the instruments than standard LRP. But the most important factor in the success of either type of LRP is the surgeon's experience, commitment, and skill.

Robotic LRP has been in use since 2003 in the United States. The machines themselves are expensive and are available in only a limited number of medical centers across the country. Still, this approach has become more popular in recent years. Early reports have found less blood loss and shorter recovery times compared with standard radical prostatectomy. But because robotic LRP is still a relatively new way of doing the surgery, reports of long-term outcomes are not yet available.

If you are thinking about treatment with either type of laparoscopic procedure, it is important to understand what is known and what is not yet known about this approach. Again, the most important factors are likely to be the skill and experience of your surgeon. If you decide that LRP is the treatment for you, be sure to find a surgeon with a lot of experience doing LRP.

Transurethral resection of the prostate

Transurethral resection of the prostate (TURP) is more commonly used to treat men with benign prostatic hyperplasia (BPH), noncancerous enlargement of the prostate. When used for prostate cancer treatment, TURP is considered a palliative approach, which means it is done to relieve symptoms, not for cure. This surgery may be used if you are having trouble urinating because of the cancer.

During TURP, the surgeon removes the inner part of the prostate gland that surrounds the urethra (the tube through which urine exits the bladder). The skin is not cut with this surgery. An instrument called a **resectoscope** is passed through the end of the penis into the urethra to the level of the prostate. Once it is in place, electricity is passed through a wire to heat it and cut or vaporize the tissue. Either spinal anesthesia (which numbs the lower half of the body) or general anesthesia (during which the patient is asleep) is used.

The operation usually takes about an hour. After surgery, a catheter is inserted through the penis into the bladder. It remains in place for 1 to 3 days to help urine drain while the prostate heals. The patient can usually leave the hospital after 1 to 2 days and return to work in 1 to 2 weeks. There will likely be some blood in the urine after surgery. Other side effects from TURP include infection and any risks that come with the type of anesthesia that is used.

Surgical risks of radical prostatectomy (including LRP)

There are possible risks with any type of surgery for prostate cancer.

Surgical risks: The risks with any type of radical prostatectomy are much like those of any major surgery, including risks from anesthesia.

Among the most serious, there is a small risk of heart attack, stroke, blood clots in the legs that may travel to the lungs, and infection at the incision site. Because there are many blood vessels near the prostate gland, another risk is bleeding during and after the surgery. You may need blood transfusions, which carry their own small risk. In extremely rare cases, people die of complications from this operation. Your risk depends, in part, on your overall health, your age, and the skill of your surgical team.

Side effects: The major possible side effects of radical prostatectomy are urinary **incontinence** (being unable to control urine) and impotence (being unable to have erections). It should be noted that these side effects are also possible with other forms of therapy, although they are described here in more detail.

Urinary incontinence: Urinary incontinence is not being able to control your urine or to have leakage or dribbling. There are different degrees of incontinence. Being incontinent can affect you not only physically but emotionally and socially as well. There are 3 major types of incontinence: stress incontinence, overflow incontinence, and urge incontinence.

- Men with **stress incontinence** leak urine when they cough, laugh, sneeze, or exercise. Stress incontinence is usually caused by problems with the bladder sphincter, the muscular valve that keeps urine in the bladder. Prostate cancer treatments may damage the muscles that form this valve or the nerves that keep the muscles working. Stress incontinence is the most common type of incontinence after prostate surgery.

- Men with **overflow incontinence** cannot empty the bladder well. They take a long time to urinate and have a dribbling stream with little force. Overflow incontinence is usually caused by blockage or narrowing of the bladder outlet by cancer or scar tissue.
- Men with **urge incontinence** have a sudden need to go to the bathroom and pass urine. This problem occurs when the bladder becomes too sensitive to stretching as urine fills it.

Rarely after surgery, men lose all ability to control their urine. This condition is called continuous incontinence.

For men who have had surgery for prostate cancer, normal bladder control usually returns within several weeks or months after radical prostatectomy. This recovery usually occurs gradually, in stages.

Doctors can't predict how any man will function after surgery. In one study of 901 men aged 55 to 74 who were treated in all different types of hospitals, researchers found the following conclusions 5 years after radical prostatectomy:

- 15% of the 901 men had no bladder control or had frequent leaks or dripping of urine.
- 16% leaked at least twice a day.

- 29% wore pads to keep dry. (Some of the men were in 2 or 3 of these groups, so adding these percentages together overstates the likelihood of urinary problems.)

Fewer problems with incontinence are reported from most large cancer centers, where prostate surgery is done more often and surgeons have more experience.

Treatment of incontinence depends on its type, cause, and severity. If you have problems with incontinence, let your doctors know. You might feel embarrassed about discussing this issue, but remember that you are not alone. This is a common problem. Doctors who treat men with prostate cancer should know about incontinence and be able to suggest ways to improve it such as these:

- Special exercises called **Kegel exercises** can help strengthen your bladder muscles. These exercises involve tensing and relaxing certain pelvic muscles. Not all doctors agree about their usefulness or the best way to do them, so ask your doctor about doing Kegel exercises before you try them.
- Medication to help the muscles of the bladder or sphincter. Most of these medicines affect either the muscles or the nerves that control them. These medicines are more effective for some forms of incontinence such as urge incontinence, than for others.
- Surgery may also be used to correct long-term incontinence. Material such

as collagen can be injected to tighten the bladder sphincter. If your incontinence is severe and not getting better on its own, an **artificial sphincter** can be implanted, or a small device called a urethral sling may be implanted to keep the bladder neck where it belongs. Ask your doctor if these treatments might help you.

Even if your incontinence cannot be completely corrected, it can still be helped. You can learn how to manage and live with your incontinence. Incontinence is more than a physical problem. It can disrupt your quality of life if it is not managed well.

There is no one right way to cope with incontinence. The challenge is to find what works for you so that you can return to your normal daily activities. There are many incontinence products to help keep you mobile and comfortable, such as pads that are worn under your clothing. Adult briefs and undergarments are bulkier than pads but provide more protection. Bed pads or absorbent mattress covers can also be used to protect the bed linens and mattress.

When choosing incontinence products, keep in mind the checklist below. Some of these questions may not be important to you, or you may have others to add.

Absorbency: How much does the product provide? How long will it protect?

Bulk: Can it be seen under normal clothing? Is it disposable? Reusable?

Comfort: How does it feel when you move or sit down?

Availability: Which stores carry the product? Are they easy to get to?

Cost: Does your insurance pay for these products?

Another option is a rubber sheath called a condom catheter that can be put over the penis to collect urine in a bag. There are also compression (pressure) devices that can be placed on the penis for short periods of time to keep urine from coming out.

For some types of incontinence, self-catheterization may be an option. In this approach, you insert a thin tube into your urethra to drain and empty the bladder. Most people can learn this safe and usually painless technique.

You can also follow some simple precautions that may make incontinence less of a problem. For example, empty your bladder before bedtime or before strenuous activity. Avoid drinking too much fluid, particularly if the drinks contain caffeine or alcohol, which can make you have to go more often. Because fat in the abdomen can push on the bladder, losing weight sometimes helps improve bladder control.

Fear, anxiety, and anger are common feelings for people dealing with incontinence. Fear of having an accident may keep you from doing the things you enjoy most—taking your grandchild to the park, going to the movies, or playing a round of golf. You may feel isolated and embarrassed.

You may even avoid sex because you are afraid of leakage. Be sure and talk to your doctor so you can begin to manage this problem.

Impotence: Impotence, also known as **erectile dysfunction**, means you cannot get an erection sufficient for sexual penetration. The nerves that allow men to get erections may be damaged or removed by radical prostatectomy. Other treatments (besides surgery) may also damage these nerves or the blood vessels that supply blood to the penis to cause an erection.

Recovering sexual function can take up to 2 years after surgery. During the first several months, you will probably not be able to have a spontaneous erection, so you may need to use medicines or other treatments. Your ability to have an erection after surgery depends on your age, your ability to get an erection before the operation, and whether the nerves were cut. Everyone can expect some decrease in the ability to have an erection, but the younger you are, the more likely it is that you will keep this ability.

There is a wide range of impotency rates reported in the medical literature. Some cancer centers that perform many radical nerve-sparing prostatectomies report impotence rates as low as 25% to 30% for men under 60, and as low as 10% for men under 50. However, other doctors have reported higher rates of impotence in similar patients. Impotence occurs in about 70% to 80% of men over 70, even if nerves on both sides are not removed.

If potency remains after surgery, the sensation of orgasm should continue to be pleasurable. There, however, will be no ejaculation of semen during orgasm. The orgasm will be "dry" because, during the prostatectomy, the glands that made most of the fluid for semen (the seminal vesicles and prostate) were removed, and the **vas deferens**, the pathways used by sperm, were cut.

Most doctors believe that regaining potency is helped along by attempting to get an erection as soon as possible once the body has had a chance to heal (usually about 6 weeks after the operation). Medicines (see below) may be helpful at this time. Be sure to talk to your doctor about your situation.

Several options may help you if you have erectile dysfunction:

- **Phosphodiesterase inhibitors,** such as sildenafil (Viagra), vardenafil (Levitra), and tadalafil (Cialis), are pills that can promote erections. These drugs will not work if both nerves have been damaged or removed. The most common side effects are headache, flushing (skin becomes red and feels warm), upset stomach, light sensitivity, and runny or stuffy nose. Nitrates, drugs used to treat heart disease, can interact with phosphodiesterase inhibitors to cause very low blood pressure, which can be dangerous. Some other drugs may also cause problems, so be sure your doctor knows which medicines you are taking.

  Some studies have found that phosphodiesterase inhibitors may, in very rare cases, block blood flow to the optic nerve in the back of the eye. This blockage could lead to blindness. Men with this complication often have had a history of smoking or problems with high blood pressure, diabetes, or high levels of cholesterol or fat in their blood.

- **Prostaglandin E1** is a substance naturally made in the body that can produce erections. A man-made version of this substance (alprostadil) can be injected almost painlessly into the base of the penis 5 to 10 minutes before intercourse or introduced into the tip of the penis as a suppository. You can even increase the dosage to prolong the erection. You may have side effects, such as pain, dizziness, and prolonged erection, but they are usually minimal.

- A **vacuum pump** is another option that may create an erection. These mechanical pumps are placed around the entire penis before intercourse to produce an erection.

- A **penile implant** might restore your ability to have erections if other methods do not help. An operation is needed to put them in place. There are several types of penile implants, including those using silicone rods or inflatable devices.

For more detailed information on coping with erection problems and other sexuality issues, contact your American Cancer Society at **800-227-2345** and request the document *Sexuality and Cancer: For the Man Who Has Cancer and His Partner* or visit our Web site, **cancer.org**.

Changes in orgasm: This can be a side effect of prostatectomy. In some men, orgasm becomes less intense or goes away completely. A few men report pain with orgasm.

Sterility: Radical prostatectomy cuts the connection between the testicles (where sperm are produced) and the urethra. This means that a man can no longer father a child by natural means after undergoing this procedure. Often, this concern is not an issue, as men with prostate cancer tend to be older. But if sterility is a concern for you, you may want to speak with your doctor about "banking" your sperm before the operation.

Lymphedema: A rare but possible complication of removing many of the lymph nodes around the prostate is a condition called **lymphedema**. Lymph nodes normally provide a way for fluid to return from all areas of the body to the heart. When nodes are removed, fluid may collect in the legs or genital region over time, causing swelling and pain. Lymphedema can usually be treated with physical therapy, although it may not disappear completely.

Change in penis length: A possible minor effect of surgery is a decrease in penis length. In one study, about 1 out of 5 men had a 15% or greater decrease in the length of their penis.

Inguinal hernia: A prostatectomy also increases the chance of needing an inguinal (groin) hernia repair in the future. In one study, the risk was 1 in 6 within 10 years of having the surgery.

Radiation Therapy

Radiation therapy uses high-energy rays or particles to kill cancer cells. Radiation is sometimes used as the initial treatment for low-grade cancer that is still confined within the prostate gland or that has only spread to nearby tissue. Cure rates for men with these types of cancers are much like those for men getting radical prostatectomy. Radiation is also sometimes used if the cancer is not completely removed or comes back (recurs) in the area of the prostate after surgery. If the disease is more advanced, radiation may be used to reduce the size of the tumor and to provide relief from present and possible future symptoms.

Two main types of radiation therapy are used: external beam radiation and brachytherapy (internal radiation). Both appear to be good methods of treating prostate cancer, although there is more long-term information about the results of treatment with external beam radiation.

External beam radiation therapy

In **external beam radiation therapy (EBRT)**, the radiation is focused on the prostate gland from a source outside your body. It is much like getting an x-ray, but for a longer time. Before treatments start, imaging tests such as MRIs, CT scans, or plain x-rays of the pelvis are done to find the exact location of your prostate gland. The radiation team may then make some ink marks on your skin that they will use later as a guide to focus the radiation in the right area. You will usually be treated 5 days per week in an outpatient center over a period of 7 to 9 weeks. Each treatment lasts only a few minutes and is painless.

Aside from being used as a treatment for early-stage cancer, external beam radiation can also be used to help relieve bone pain when the cancer has spread to a specific area of bone.

Standard (conventional) EBRT is used much less often than in the past. Newer techniques allow doctors to give higher doses of radiation to the prostate gland while reducing the radiation exposure to nearby healthy tissues. These techniques have fewer side effects than standard EBRT. They may also have a better chance of curing the cancer, but this has not yet been proved in clinical studies.

Three-dimensional conformal radiation therapy

Three-dimensional conformal radiation therapy (3D-CRT) uses special computers to precisely map the location of your prostate. You will likely be fitted with a plastic mold resembling a body cast to keep you in the same position so that the radiation can be aimed more accurately. Radiation beams are then shaped and aimed at the prostate from several directions, which makes it less likely to damage normal tissues.

The 3D-CRT method seems to be at least as effective as standard radiation therapy, with lower side effects. Many doctors now recommend using it when it is available. In theory, by aiming the radiation more accurately, doctors can reduce radiation damage to tissues near the prostate and cure more cancers by increasing the radiation dose to the prostate. Long-term study results are still needed to confirm this theory.

Intensity modulated radiation therapy

An advanced form of 3D therapy, **intensity modulated radiation therapy (IMRT)** uses a computer-driven machine that actually moves around the patient as it delivers radiation. In addition to shaping the beams and aiming them at the prostate from several angles, the intensity (strength) of the beams can be adjusted to minimize the dose reaching the most sensitive normal tissues. This approach allows doctors to deliver an even higher dose to the cancer areas. Many major hospitals and cancer centers are now able to provide IMRT. The RapidArc™ is a form of IMRT that allows each treatment to be given over just a few minutes. It is more convenient for the patient, but is similar to regular IMRT in terms of effectiveness.

Conformal proton beam radiation therapy

Proton beam radiation therapy is related to 3D-CRT and uses a similar approach. But instead of using x-rays, this technique focuses proton beams on the cancer. Protons are positive parts of atoms. Unlike x-rays, which release energy both before and after they hit their target, protons cause little damage to tissues they pass through and then release their energy after traveling a certain distance. This means that proton beam radiation may be able to deliver more radiation to the prostate and do less damage to nearby normal tissues. As with 3D-CRT and IMRT, early results are promising, but more studies will be needed to determine whether proton beam therapy is better in the long run than standard external beam radiation. Right now, proton beam therapy is not widely available. The machines needed to make protons are expensive, and there are only a handful of them in use in the United States. Proton beam radiation may not be covered by all insurance companies at this time.

Stereotactic radiosurgery

Stereotactic radiosurgery is a form of IMRT that is most commonly used to treat cancer that spreads to the brain. It involves holding the head in a metal frame or cage to prevent any movement, while the machine delivers radiation precisely to the tumor. When only a single treatment is given, it is called stereotactic radiosurgery, but when many treatments are given it is called stereotactic radiotherapy. This treatment often goes by the names of the machines used to give it, such as Gamma Knife™, Novalis Tx™, and CyberKnife™.

Possible side effects of external beam radiation therapy

The numbers used to describe the possible side effects below relate to standard external beam radiation therapy, which is now used much less often than in the past. The risks associated with the newer treatment methods described above are likely to be lower.

Bowel problems: During and after treatment with external beam radiation therapy, there may be diarrhea, sometimes with blood in the stool, rectal leakage, and an irritated large intestine. Most of these problems go away over time, but in rare cases normal bowel function does not return after treatment ends. In the past, about 10% to 20% of men reported bowel problems after external beam radiation therapy, but the newer conformal radiation techniques may be less likely to cause these problems.

Bladder problems: A patient may need to urinate more frequently and may experience a burning sensation while urinating, and there may be blood in the urine. Bladder problems usually improve over time but, in some patients, they never go away. About 1 patient in 3 continues to have problems with needing to urinate more often.

Urinary incontinence: Urinary incontinence is less common after radiation than after surgery overall, but the chance of incontinence goes up each year for several years after radiation treatment.

Impotence: After a few years, the impotence rate after external beam radiation therapy is about the same as that after surgery. Impotence usually does not occur right after radiation therapy, but impotence slowly develops over a year or more. This contrasts with the side effects from surgery, where impotence occurs immediately and may improve over time. In older studies, about 3 out of 4 men were impotent within 5 years of having external beam radiation therapy (some of these men had erection problems before treatment). In men who had normal erections before treatment, about half became impotent at 5 years. It is unclear whether these numbers will apply to newer forms of radiation as well. As with surgery, however, the older the patient is, the more likely he will become impotent. Impotence may be helped by treatments such as those listed on pages 75–76, including erectile dysfunction medicines.

Fatigue: Radiation therapy may also cause **fatigue** (feeling tired) that may not disappear until a few months after treatment stops.

Lymphedema: Fluid buildup in the legs or genitals, a condition called lymphedema (described in the surgery section on page 77), is possible if the lymph nodes receive radiation.

Brachytherapy (Internal Radiation Therapy)

Brachytherapy (also called seed implantation or **interstitial radiation therapy**) uses small radioactive pellets, or "seeds," each about the size of a grain of rice. These pellets are placed directly into the prostate. Brachytherapy is generally used only in men with early-stage prostate cancer that is relatively slow growing.

Use of brachytherapy may also be limited by other factors. For men who have had a transurethral resection of the prostate (TURP) or for those who already have urinary problems, the risk of urinary side effects may be higher. Brachytherapy may not be as effective in men with large prostate glands because many more seeds may be needed. Doctors are now looking at ways to avoid this problem, such as giving men a short course of hormone therapy beforehand to shrink the prostate.

Imaging tests such as transrectal ultrasound, CT scans, or MRI help guide the placement of the radioactive pellets. Special computer programs calculate the exact dose of radiation needed. Without these calculations, the cancer might get too little radiation or the normal tissues around it could get too much.

There are 2 types of prostate brachytherapy. Both are done in an operating room and require some type of anesthesia.

Permanent (low dose rate) brachytherapy

With permanent (low dose rate, or LDR) brachytherapy, pellets (seeds) of radioactive material (such as iodine-125 or palladium-103) are placed inside thin needles, which are inserted through the skin in the area between the scrotum and anus (perineum) and into the prostate. The pellets are left in place as the needles are removed and give off low doses of radiation for weeks or months. Radiation from the seeds travels a very short distance, so the seeds can put out a very large amount of radiation to a very small area. This decreases the amount of damage done to the healthy tissues that are close to the prostate.

Usually, 40 to 100 seeds are placed. Because they are so small, their presence causes little discomfort, and they are simply left in place after their radioactive material is used up. This type of radiation therapy requires spinal anesthesia (where the lower half of your body is numbed) or general anesthesia (where you are asleep) and may require 1 day in the hospital.

You may also receive external beam radiation along with brachytherapy, especially if there is a risk that your cancer has spread outside of the prostate (for example, if you have a high Gleason score).

Temporary (high dose rate) brachytherapy

Temporary or **high dose rate (HDR) brachytherapy** is a newer technique in which hollow needles are placed through the perineum into the prostate. Soft nylon tubes (catheters) are placed in these needles. The needles are then removed but the catheters stay in place. Radioactive iridium-192 or cesium-137 is then placed in the catheters, usually for 5 to 15 minutes. Generally, about 3 brief treatments are given, and the radioactive substance is removed each time. The treatments are usually given over a couple of days. After the last treatment, the catheters are removed. For about a week following placement of the catheters, you may have some pain in the area between your scrotum and rectum, and your urine may be reddish-brown.

High-dose radiation treatments are usually combined with external beam radiation given at a lower dose than when used alone. The total dose of radiation is computed so that it is high enough to kill all the cancer cells. The advantage of this approach is that most of the radiation is concentrated in the prostate gland itself, sparing the urethra and the tissues around the prostate such as the nerves, bladder, and rectum.

Possible risks and side effects of brachytherapy

If you receive permanent brachytherapy seeds, they will give off small amounts of radiation for several weeks. Even though the radiation doesn't travel far, your doctor may advise you to stay away from pregnant women and small children during this time. You may be asked to take other precautions as well, such as wearing a condom during sex.

There is also a small risk that some of the seeds may move (migrate). You may be asked to strain your urine for the first week or so to catch any seeds that might come out. Be sure to carefully follow any instructions your doctor gives you. There have also been reports of the seeds moving through the bloodstream to other parts of the body, such as the lungs. As far as doctors can tell, this doesn't seem to cause any ill effects and happens very rarely.

Like external beam radiation, brachytherapy can also cause impotence, urinary problems, and bowel problems.

Bowel problems: Significant long-term bowel problems (including burning and rectal pain and/or diarrhea) occur in less than 5% of patients.

Urinary problems: Severe urinary incontinence is not a common side effect. But frequent urination may persist in about 1 of 3 patients who have brachytherapy. This reaction is perhaps caused by irritation of the urethra, the tube that drains urine from the bladder. In rare cases, this tube may actually close off (known as **urethral stricture**) and need to be opened with surgery.

Impotence: Problems with erections may be less likely to develop after brachytherapy than after other common forms of treatment, but this area of research is unclear. Some studies have found rates of sexual dysfunction to be lower after brachytherapy, but other studies have found that the impotence rates were no lower than with external beam radiation or surgery. Again, the younger you are and the better your sexual function before treatment, the more likely you will be to regain function after treatment.

Cryosurgery

Cryosurgery (also called cryotherapy or **cryoablation**) is sometimes used to treat localized prostate cancer by freezing it. As with brachytherapy, this choice may not be a good option for men with large prostate glands.

With cryosurgery, several hollow probes (needles) are placed through the skin between the anus and scrotum (the perineum). The doctor guides them into the prostate by using transrectal ultrasound (TRUS). Very cold gases are passed through the needles, creating ice balls that destroy the prostate gland. To be certain that the prostate cancer cells are destroyed without too much damage to nearby tissues, the doctor carefully watches the ultrasound images during the procedure. Warm saltwater is circulated through a catheter in the urethra to keep it from freezing. Spinal, epidural, or general anesthesia is used during the procedure.

Before cryosurgery, a suprapubic catheter is placed through a skin incision on the abdomen and into the bladder so that if the prostate swells after the procedure (which usually occurs), urine can be drained through this tube. The catheter is removed a couple of weeks later, once the swelling goes down. After the procedure, there will be some bruising and soreness in the perineum where the probes were inserted. The patient may need to stay in the hospital for a day, but many patients can leave the same day.

Cryosurgery is less invasive than radical prostatectomy, so there is usually less blood loss, a shorter hospital stay, shorter recovery period, and less pain than with surgery. But compared with surgery or radiation therapy, doctors know much less about the long-term effectiveness of cryosurgery. Current techniques using ultrasound guidance and precise temperature monitoring have only been available for a few years. Outcomes of long-term (10- to 15-year) follow-up must still be collected and reviewed. For this reason, most doctors do not often use cryotherapy as the first treatment of prostate cancer. It is sometimes recommended if the cancer has come back after other treatments.

Possible side effects of cryosurgery

Side effects from cryosurgery tend to be worse in men who have already had radiation therapy, as opposed to men who have cryosurgery as the first form of treatment.

Most men have blood in their urine for a day or two after the procedure, as well as soreness in the area where the needles were placed. Swelling of the penis or scrotum is also common. The freezing may also affect the bladder and intestines, which can lead to pain, burning sensations, and the need to empty the bladder and bowels often. Most men recover normal bowel and bladder function over time.

Freezing damages nerves near the prostate and causes impotence in up to 80% of men who have cryosurgery. Erectile dysfunction is more common after cryosurgery than after radical prostatectomy.

Urinary incontinence is rare in men who have cryosurgery as their first treatment for prostate cancer, but it is more common in men who have already had radiation therapy.

A fistula (an abnormal connection) between the rectum and bladder develops in less than 1% of men after cryosurgery. This rare but serious problem can allow urine to leak into the rectum and may require surgery to repair.

Hormone (Androgen Deprivation) Therapy

Hormone therapy is also called **androgen deprivation therapy (ADT)** or androgen suppression therapy. The goal is to reduce levels of the male hormones, called androgens, in the body. The main androgens are testosterone and dihydrotestosterone (DHT). Androgens, produced mainly in the testicles, stimulate prostate cancer cells to grow. Lowering androgen levels often makes prostate cancers shrink or grow more slowly. However, hormone therapy does not cure prostate cancer.

Hormone therapy may be used in several situations:

- if you are not able to have surgery or radiation or can't be cured by these treatments because the cancer has already spread beyond the prostate gland
- if your cancer remains or comes back after treatment with surgery or radiation therapy
- as an addition to radiation therapy as initial treatment if you are at high risk for cancer recurrence
- before surgery or radiation to try and shrink the cancer to make other treatments more effective

Types of hormone therapy

There are several types of hormone therapy used to treat prostate cancer.

Orchiectomy (surgical **castration**): Even though this is a type of surgery, it is mainly considered to be a form of hormone therapy. In this operation, the surgeon removes the testicles, where more than 90% of the androgens, mostly testosterone, are made. With this source removed, most prostate cancers stop growing or shrink for a time.

Orchiectomy is done as a simple outpatient procedure. It is probably the least expensive and simplest way to reduce androgen levels in the body. But unlike some of the other methods of lowering androgen levels, it is permanent, and many men have trouble accepting the removal of their testicles. Some men having the procedure are concerned about how it will look. If wanted, artificial silicone sacs that look much like testicles can be inserted into the scrotum.

Luteinizing hormone-releasing hormone (LHRH) analogs: Even though **LHRH analogs** (also called LHRH agonists) cost more and require more frequent doctor visits, most men choose this method over orchiectomy. These drugs lower the amount of testosterone made by the testicles. Treatment with these drugs is sometimes called **chemical castration** because they are just as effective as orchiectomy for lowering androgen levels.

LHRH analogs are injected or placed as small implants under the skin. Depending on the drug used, they are given anywhere from every month, every 3 or 4 months, up to once a year. The LHRH analogs available in the United States include leuprolide (Lupron, Viadur, Eligard), goserelin (Zoladex), triptorelin (Trelstar), and histrelin (Vantas).

When LHRH analogs are first given, testosterone production increases briefly before falling to very low levels. This effect is called flare and results from the complex way in which LHRH analogs work. Men whose cancer has spread to the bones may experience bone pain. If the cancer has spread to the spine, it could compress the spinal cord and cause pain or paralysis. Flare can be avoided by giving drugs called **antiandrogens** for a few weeks when starting treatment with LHRH analogs. (For more on antiandrogens, see page 93.)

Luteinizing hormone-releasing hormone (LHRH) antagonists: Abarelix (Plenaxis) was introduced as a newer type of drug known as an LHRH antagonist. It is believed to work like LHRH analogs, except that it appears to reduce testosterone levels more quickly and does not cause tumor flare like the LHRH analogs.

In 2005, the company making abarelix took it off the market. At that time, men who were already taking abarelix were allowed to continue taking the drug, but it could not be prescribed for new patients. It is no longer available.

Degarelix (Firmagon) is a new LHRH antagonist that was approved for use by the **U.S. Food and Drug Administration (FDA)** in 2008 to treat advanced prostate cancer. It is given as a monthly injection under the skin. Like abarelix, degarelix quickly reduces testosterone levels. In early studies, the most common side effects shown with this drug were problems at the injection site (pain, redness, and swelling) and increased levels of liver enzymes on laboratory tests. Other side effects are discussed in detail in the next section.

Antiandrogens: Antiandrogens block the body's ability to use any androgens. Even after orchiectomy or during treatment with LHRH analogs, androgens are still produced in small amounts by the adrenal glands.

Antiandrogens such as flutamide (Eulexin), bicalutamide (Casodex), and nilutamide (Nilandron) are taken daily in pill form.

Antiandrogens are not often used alone. An antiandrogen may be added when treatment with orchiectomy or with an LHRH analog, for example, is no longer working. An antiandrogen is sometimes given for a few weeks when an LHRH analog is first started to prevent a tumor flare (see page 92).

Antiandrogen treatment may be combined with orchiectomy or LHRH analogs as first-line hormone therapy. This is called **combined androgen blockade**. There is still some debate as to whether combined androgen blockade is more effective in this setting than using orchiectomy or an LHRH analog alone. If there is a benefit, it appears to be small.

Some doctors are testing the use of antiandrogens *instead of* orchiectomy or LHRH analogs. Several recent studies have compared the effectiveness of antiandrogens alone with that of LHRH analogs. Most studies have shown no difference in survival rates, but a few studies showed antiandrogens to be slightly less effective.

If hormone therapy, including an antiandrogen, stops working, some men seem to benefit for a short time from simply stopping the antiandrogen. Doctors call this the "antiandrogen withdrawal" effect, although they are not sure why it happens.

Other androgen-suppressing drugs: Estrogens were once the main alternative to orchiectomy for men with advanced prostate cancer. Because of their possible side effects (including blood clots and breast enlargement), estrogens have been largely replaced by LHRH analogs and antiandrogens. Still, estrogens may be tried if androgen deprivation is no longer working.

Ketoconazole (Nizoral), first used for treating fungal infections, blocks production of androgens and is sometimes used in prostate cancer treatment. It can also block the production of cortisol in the body. People treated with ketoconozole often need to take a corticosteroid (like hydrocortisone) along with it in order to prevent the side effects caused by low cortisol levels.

Side effects of hormone therapy

Orchiectomy, LHRH analogs (or agonists), and LHRH antagonists all cause side effects due to changes in the levels of hormones such as testosterone and estrogen. These side effects can include the following:

- reduced or absent libido (sexual desire)
- impotence
- hot flashes (these may get better or even go away with time)
- breast tenderness and growth of breast tissue
- osteoporosis (bone thinning), which can lead to broken bones
- anemia (low red blood cell counts)
- decreased mental acuity (sharpness)
- loss of muscle mass
- weight gain
- fatigue
- increased cholesterol
- depression

The risk of hypertension (high blood pressure), diabetes, and heart attacks (myocardial infarctions) is also higher in men treated with hormone therapy.

Antiandrogens have similar side effects. The major difference from LHRH analogs and orchiectomy is that antiandrogens may have fewer sexual side effects. When these drugs are used alone, libido and potency can often be maintained. When these drugs are given to patients already being treated with LHRH analogs, diarrhea is the major side effect. Nausea, liver problems, and tiredness can also occur.

Many side effects can be prevented or treated. For example, hot flashes can be helped by treatment with certain antidepressants. Brief radiation treatment to the breasts can help prevent their enlargement. There are several different drugs available to prevent and treat osteoporosis. Depression can be treated by antidepressants and/or counseling. Exercise can help reduce many side effects, including fatigue, weight gain, and the chance of loss of bone and muscle mass. If anemia occurs, it is often very mild and usually doesn't cause symptoms.

There is growing concern that hormone therapy for prostate cancer may have a negative effect on cognition—it may lead to problems with thinking, concentration, and/or memory. A number of studies have examined the link between testosterone levels and brain function, first in animals, then in healthy men. But this link has not been studied well in men getting hormone therapy for prostate cancer. The studies that have been done are small and often had conflicting results. Different studies have shown changes in different types of memory. Some have even found that while some types of memory get worse, another type got better. Other studies found no effect at all.

Studying the effect of hormone therapy on brain function is difficult, because other factors may also change the way the brain works. A study has to take all of these factors into account. For example, age is an issue. Both prostate cancer and memory problems become more common as people get older. Also, hormone therapy can lead to anemia, fatigue, and depression—all of which can affect brain function. Still, hormone therapy does seem to lead to memory problems in some patients. These problems are rarely severe, and most often affect only some types of memory. More studies are being done to look at this issue.

Current controversies in hormone therapy

There are many issues around hormone therapy that not all doctors agree on, such as the best time to start and stop it and the best way to give it. Studies looking at these issues are now under way. A few of the issues are discussed here.

Treating early stage cancer: Some men with early (stage I or II) prostate cancer have been treated with hormone therapy instead of surgery or radiation. A recent study found that these men do not live any longer than those who did not receive any treatment at first, but instead waited until the cancer progressed or symptoms developed.

Early versus delayed treatment: Some doctors believe that hormone therapy works better if it is started as soon as possible, even though the patient feels well. This applies to cancer in an advanced stage (for example, when it has spread to lymph nodes), a tumor that is large (T3) or has a high Gleason score, or when the PSA levels have begun to rise after the initial therapy. Some studies have shown that hormone treatment may slow down the disease and perhaps even lengthen patient survival. But not all doctors agree with this approach. Some are waiting for more evidence of benefit. Because of the likely side effects and the chance that the cancer could become resistant to therapy sooner, they believe that treatment should not be started until symptoms from the disease appear. Studies addressing these questions are now under way.

Intermittent versus continuous hormone therapy: Nearly all prostate cancers treated with hormone therapy become resistant to this treatment over a period of months or years. Some doctors believe that constant androgen suppression may not be needed, so they advise intermittent (on-again, off-again) treatment.

In one form of intermittent therapy, androgen suppression is stopped once the blood PSA level drops to a very low level. If the PSA level begins to rise, the drugs are started again. Another form of intermittent therapy involves using androgen suppression for fixed periods—for example, 6 months on, followed by 6 months off.

Clinical trials of **intermittent hormone therapy** are still in progress. It is too early to say whether this new approach is better or worse than continuous hormone therapy. However, one advantage of intermittent treatment is that for a while some men are able to avoid the side effects of hormone therapy such as impotence, hot flashes, and loss of sex drive.

Combined androgen blockade (CAB): Some doctors treat patients with both androgen deprivation (orchiectomy or an LHRH analog) and an antiandrogen. A recent study found that men who received CAB in addition to radiation treatments were less likely to die of prostate cancer than those who received an LHRH analog with radiation. Another study that looked at men with metastatic prostate cancer found that those treated with CAB lived longer than those treated with an LHRH analog alone. But most doctors are not convinced there's enough evidence that this combined therapy is better than one drug alone when treating metastatic prostate cancer.

Triple androgen blockade (TAB): Some doctors have suggested taking combined therapy one step further, by adding a drug called a 5 alpha-reductase inhibitor—either finasteride (Proscar, Propecia) or dutasteride (Avodart)—to the combined androgen blockade. There is currently very little evidence to support the use of this "triple androgen blockade" approach.

Chemotherapy

Chemotherapy is sometimes used if prostate cancer has spread outside of the prostate gland and hormone therapy is not working. Chemotherapy is not a standard treatment for early prostate cancer, but some studies are examining whether it could be helpful when administered for a short time after surgery.

Chemotherapy involves the use of anticancer drugs, which are injected into a vein or given by mouth. These drugs enter the bloodstream and go throughout the body, making this treatment potentially useful for cancers that have spread (metastasized) to distant organs.

At one time, chemotherapy was not believed to be very effective in treating prostate cancer, but this has changed in recent years. A combination of the chemotherapy drug docetaxel (Taxotere) and the steroid drug prednisone has been shown to reduce symptoms and prolong life (when compared with other chemotherapy drugs) in patients with advanced prostate cancer. Most doctors now consider this to be the first-line chemotherapy option in men whose cancer is no longer responding to hormonal treatments. Recently, a new drug called cabazitaxel (Jevtana) was approved for use in men with advanced prostate cancer. When given to men whose cancers had stopped responding to docetaxel, the new drug cabazitaxel helped them live longer.

Some of the other chemotherapy drugs used to treat prostate cancer include the following:

- mitoxantrone (Novantrone)
- estramustine (Emcyt)
- doxorubicin (Adriamycin)
- etoposide (VP-16)
- vinblastine (Velban)
- paclitaxel (Taxol)
- carboplatin (Paraplatin)
- vinorelbine (Navelbine)

Like hormone therapy, chemotherapy is unlikely to result in a cure. This treatment is not expected to destroy all the cancer cells, but it may slow the cancer's growth and reduce symptoms, resulting in a better quality of life.

Possible side effects of chemotherapy

Chemotherapy drugs work by attacking cells that are dividing quickly, which is why they work against cancer cells. But other cells in the body, such as those in the bone marrow, the lining of the mouth and intestines, and the hair follicles, also divide quickly. These cells are also likely to be affected by chemotherapy, which can lead to side effects.

The side effects of chemotherapy depend on the type and dose of drugs given and the length of time they are taken. These side effects may include the following:

- hair loss
- mouth sores
- loss of appetite
- nausea and vomiting
- lowered resistance to infection (due to low white blood cell counts)
- easy bruising or bleeding (due to low platelet counts)
- fatigue (due to low red blood cell counts)

In addition, each chemotherapy drug may have its own unique side effects. For example, estramustine, a drug sometimes used to treat prostate cancer, also carries the risk of blood clots. Docetaxel can cause severe allergic reactions. Medication is given before docetaxel treatments to prevent this problem. Doxorubicin can weaken the heart muscle over time, so doctors must limit the amount of this drug that is used. Although it is rare, mitoxantrone can cause leukemia, so it is no longer being studied for use in early prostate cancer.

The side effects of chemotherapy are usually short-term and go away once treatment is finished.

There is help for many of these side effects. For example, drugs can be given to prevent or reduce nausea and vomiting. Other drugs can be given to boost blood cell counts.

Vaccine Treatment

A prostate cancer vaccine, sipuleucel-T (Provenge), has recently been approved by the FDA to treat advanced prostate cancer. Unlike most vaccines, this vaccine is aimed at treating prostate cancer, not preventing it. Also, this vaccine is unique to each person who gets it—it is not mass produced.

When sipuleucel-T is administered, white blood cells (cells of the immune system) are removed from the patient's blood and exposed to a protein from prostate cancer cells called **prostatic acid phosphatase (PAP)**. These cells are then given back to the patient by infusion into a vein (IV). This process is repeated 2 more times, 2 weeks apart, so that the patient gets 3 doses of cells. In the body, the cells induce other immune system cells to attack the patient's prostate cancer. Common side effects include fever, chills, fatigue, back and joint pain, nausea, and headache. These most often start during the cell infusions and last no more than a day or 2. A few men had more severe symptoms, including problems breathing and high blood pressure, which improved with treatment. When used in men with metastatic prostate cancer that no longer responded to hormone therapy, the vaccine helped them live more than 4 months longer on average (than the men who didn't get the vaccine). Studies are continuing to determine whether this vaccine can help men with less advanced prostate cancer.

Treating Pain

Most of this book talks about ways to remove or to destroy prostate cancer cells or to slow their growth. But maintaining your quality of life is another important goal. Don't hesitate to discuss pain, other symptoms, or any quality of life concerns with your cancer care team. Pain and most other symptoms of prostate cancer can often be treated effectively. If the treatments listed above don't help with symptoms, there are several other options.

Pain medicines

When properly prescribed, pain medicines (ranging from aspirin to opioids) are very effective. You may worry about addiction or dependence with opioids, but this is almost never a problem if the drug is being used as directed to treat cancer pain. Symptoms such as drowsiness and constipation are possible but can usually be treated by changing the dose or by adding other medicines.

Bisphosphonates: Bisphosphonates are a group of drugs that can help relieve bone pain caused by cancer that has spread (metastasized). These drugs may also slow the growth of the metastases and prevent fractures. **Bisphosphonates** also help to strengthen bones in men who are also receiving hormone therapy. The most commonly used bisphosphonate is zoledronic acid (Zometa), which is approved for use in bone metastases from prostate cancer. It is given as an intravenous (IV) injection. Other bisphosphonates have been approved for other uses, and some doctors use these "off label" (to treat a condition for which the drugs have not been approved by the U.S. Food and Drug Administration) to treat prostate cancer.

Bisphosphonates can have their own side effects, including flu-like symptoms and bone pain. A rare but very distressing side effect of bisphosphonates is something called osteonecrosis of the jaw bone. With this condition, the blood supply to an area in the bone stops, and that part of the bone dies. This can lead to tooth loss and infections or open sores of the jaw bone that won't heal. There is no really good way to treat this condition, other than to stop the drug and give supportive care. Doctors don't know why some people experience jaw osteonecrosis while on bisphosphonates, but it seems to occur more frequently after dental work (such as having a tooth pulled) is done while on this medicine. That is why many cancer doctors recommend that patients who will be starting a bisphosphonate have a dental checkup so that any tooth or jaw problems can be treated before they start taking the drug. Maintaining good oral hygiene by flossing and brushing, making sure that dentures fit properly, and having regular dental checkups may also help prevent this condition.

Steroids: Some studies suggest that corticosteroids (such as prednisone and dexamethasone) can help relieve bone pain in some men.

External radiation therapy

Radiation therapy can help reduce bone pain, especially if the pain is limited to one or only a few areas of bone. Radiation can be aimed at tumors on the spine, which can help relieve pressure on the spinal cord in some cases. Radiation therapy may also help relieve other symptoms by shrinking tumors in other parts of the body.

Radiopharmaceuticals: Strontium-89 (Metastron) and Samarium-153 (Quadramet) are drugs that contain radioactive elements. They are injected into a vein and collect in bones. Once there, the radiation they emit kills the cancer cells and relieves some of the pain caused by bone metastases. About 80% of prostate cancer patients with painful bone metastases are helped by this treatment.

Radiopharmaceuticals are used to treat bone pain caused by metastatic prostate cancer— they are not for early-stage prostate cancer. These drugs are especially helpful when prostate cancer has spread to many bones, since external beam radiation would need to be aimed at each affected bone. In some cases, one of these drugs will be used together with external beam radiation aimed at the most painful bone metastases.

The major side effect of this treatment is a lowering of blood cell counts, which could place you at increased risk for infections or bleeding, especially if your counts are already low.

It is very important that your pain be treated effectively. This treatment will help you feel better and allow you to focus on the people and activities that are most important to you.

Clinical Trials

If you have been told you have prostate cancer, you have a lot of decisions to make. One of the most important decisions you will make is deciding which treatment is best for you. You may have heard about clinical trials being done for your type of cancer. Or maybe someone on your health care team has mentioned a **clinical trial** to you. Clinical trials are one way to get state-of-the art cancer care. Still, they are not right for everyone.

Here we will give you a brief overview of clinical trials. Talking to your health care team, your family, and your friends can help you make the best treatment choices.

Clinical trials are carefully controlled research studies that are done with patients. These studies test whether a new treatment is safe and how well it works in patients, or they may test new ways to diagnose or prevent a disease. Clinical trials have led to many advances in cancer prevention, diagnosis, and treatment.

Clinical trials are done to get a closer look at promising new treatments or procedures in patients. A clinical trial is undertaken only when there is good reason to believe that the treatment, test, or procedure being studied may be better than the one already being used. Treatments used in clinical trials are often found to have real benefits and may go on to become tomorrow's standard treatment.

Clinical trials can focus on many things:

- new uses of drugs that are already approved by the U.S. Food and Drug Administration (FDA)
- new drugs that have not yet been approved by the FDA
- nondrug treatments (such as radiation therapy)
- medical procedures (such as types of surgery)
- herbs and vitamins
- tools to improve the ways medicines or diagnostic tests are used
- medicines or procedures to relieve symptoms or improve comfort
- combinations of treatments and procedures

Researchers conduct studies of new treatments to try to answer the following questions:

- Is the treatment helpful?
- What's the best way to give it?
- Does it work better than other treatments already available?
- What side effects does the treatment cause?
- Are there more or fewer side effects than the standard treatment used now?
- Do the benefits outweigh the side effects?
- In which patients is the treatment most likely to be helpful?

There are 4 phases of clinical trials, which are numbered I, II, III, and IV. We will use the example of testing a new cancer treatment drug to look at what each phase is like.

Phase I clinical trials

The purpose of a phase I study is to find the safest way to give a new treatment to patients. The cancer care team closely watches patients for any harmful side effects.

For phase I studies, the drug has already been tested in laboratory and animal studies, but the side effects in patients are not fully known. Doctors start by giving very low doses of the drug to the first patients and increase the doses for later groups of patients until side effects appear or the desired effect is seen. Doctors are hoping to help the study patients, but the main purpose of a phase I trial is to test the safety of the drug.

Phase I clinical trials are often done in small groups of people with different cancers that have not responded to standard treatment, or that recur after treatment. If a drug is found to be reasonably safe in phase I studies, it can be tested in a phase II clinical trial.

Phase II clinical trials

These studies are designed to see whether the drug is effective. Patients are given the most appropriate (safest) dose as determined from phase I studies. They are closely watched for an effect on the cancer. The cancer care team also looks for side effects. Phase II trials are often done in larger groups of patients with a specific cancer type that has not responded to standard treatment. If a drug is found to be effective in phase II studies, it can be tested in a phase III clinical trial.

Phase III clinical trials

Phase III studies involve large numbers of patients—most often those patients who have just received a diagnosis for a specific type of cancer. Phase III clinical trials may enroll thousands of patients. Often, these studies are randomized, which means that patients are randomly put in 1 of 2 (or more) groups. One group (called the control group) gets the standard, most accepted treatment. The other group(s) gets the new treatment(s) being studied. All patients in phase III studies are closely watched. The study will be stopped early if many patients have side effects from the new treatment that are too severe or if one group has much better results than the others. Phase III clinical trials are needed before the FDA will approve a treatment for use by the general public.

Phase IV clinical trials

Once a drug has been approved by the FDA and is available for all patients, it is still studied in other clinical trials (sometimes referred to as phase IV studies). This way, more can be learned about short-term and long-term side effects and safety as the drug is used in larger numbers of patients with many types of diseases. Doctors can also learn more about how well the drug works and whether it might be helpful when used in other ways (such as in combination with other treatments).

What it is like to be in a clinical trial

If you participate in a clinical trial, you will have a team of cancer care experts taking care of you and watching your progress very carefully. Depending on the phase of the clinical trial, you may receive more attention (such as having more doctor visits and laboratory tests) than you would if you were treated outside of a clinical trial. Clinical trials are designed to pay close attention to you. However, there are some risks. No one involved in the study knows in advance whether the treatment will work or exactly what side effects will occur. That outcome is what the study is designed to find out. While most side effects go away in time, some may be long-lasting or even life-threatening. Keep in mind, though, that even standard treatments have side effects.

Deciding to enter a clinical trial

If you would like to take part in a clinical trial, you should begin by asking your doctor if your clinic or hospital conducts clinical trials. There are requirements you must meet to take part in any clinical trial. But whether or not you enter (enroll in) a clinical trial is completely up to you. The doctors and nurses conducting the study will explain the study to you in detail. They will go over the possible risks and benefits and give you a form (informed consent) to read and sign. The form says that you understand the clinical trial and want to take part in it. Even after you read and sign the form and after the clinical trial begins, you are free to leave the study at any time, for any reason. Taking part in a clinical trial does not keep you from getting any other medical care you may need.

To find out more about clinical trials, talk to your cancer care team. Here are some questions you might ask:

- Is there a clinical trial that I should take part in?
- What is the purpose of the study?
- How might this study be of benefit to me?
- What is likely to happen in my case with, or without, this new treatment?
- What kinds of tests and treatments does the study involve?
- What does this treatment do? Has it been used before?
- Will I know which treatment I receive?
- What are my other choices and their pros and cons?
- How could the study affect my daily life?
- What side effects can I expect from the study? Can the side effects be controlled?
- Will I have to stay in the hospital? If so, how often and for how long?
- Will the study cost me anything? Will any of the treatment be free?
- If I am harmed as a result of the research, what treatment would I be entitled to?
- What type of long-term follow-up care is part of the study?
- Has the treatment been used to treat other types of cancer?

How can I find out more about clinical trials that might be right for me?

The American Cancer Society offers a clinical trials matching service for use by patients, their family, or friends. You can reach this service at **800-303-5691** or on the Web at **http://clinicaltrials .cancer.org**.

Based on the information you give about your cancer type, stage, and previous treatments, this service can put together a list of clinical trials that match your medical needs. The service will also ask where you live and whether you are willing to travel so that it can look for a treatment center that you can get to. You can also get a list of current clinical trials by calling the National Cancer Institute's Cancer Information Service toll-free at **800-4-CANCER** (**800-422-6237**) or by visiting the NCI clinical trials Web site at **www.cancer .gov/clinicaltrials**.

For even more information on clinical trials, see the American Cancer Society document *Clinical Trials: What You Need to Know*, available on the Web at **cancer.org**. You may also request this document by calling our toll-free number, **800-227-2345**.

Complementary and Alternative Treatments

When you have cancer, you are likely to hear about ways to treat your cancer or relieve symptoms that are different from mainstream (standard) medical treatment. These treatments can include vitamins, herbs, and special diets, or acupuncture and massage—among many others. You may have a lot of questions about these treatments. Talk to your doctor about any treatment you are considering. Here are some questions to ask:

- How do I know if the treatment is safe?
- How do I know if it works?
- Should I try one or more of these treatments?
- Will these treatments cause a problem with my standard medical treatment?
- What is the difference between complementary and alternative treatments?
- Where can I find out more about these treatments?

The terms can be confusing

Not everyone uses these terms the same way, so it can be confusing. The American Cancer Society uses **complementary medicine** to refer to medicines or treatments that are used *along with* your regular medical care. **Alternative medicine** is a treatment used *instead of* standard medical treatment.

Complementary treatments

Complementary treatment methods, for the most part, are not presented as cures for cancer. Most often they are used to help you feel better. Some methods that can be used in a complementary way are meditation to reduce stress, acupuncture to relieve pain, or peppermint tea to relieve nausea. There are many others. Some of these methods are known to help and could add to your comfort and well-being, while others have not been tested. Some have been proven not to be helpful. A few have even been found harmful. There are many complementary methods that you can safely use right along with your medical treatment to help relieve symptoms or side effects, to ease pain, and to help you enjoy life more. For example, some people find methods such as aromatherapy, massage therapy, meditation, or yoga to be useful.

Alternative treatments

Alternative treatments are those methods that are used instead of standard medical care. These treatments have not been proven to be safe and effective in clinical trials. Some of these treatments may even be dangerous or have life-threatening side effects. The biggest danger in most cases is that you may lose the chance to benefit from standard treatment. Delays or interruptions in your standard medical treatment may give the cancer more time to grow.

Deciding what to do

It is easy to see why people with cancer may consider alternative treatments. You want to do all you can to fight the cancer. Sometimes mainstream treatments such as chemotherapy can be hard to take, or they may no longer be working. Sometimes people suggest that their treatment can cure your cancer without having serious side effects, and it's normal to want to believe them. But the truth is that most nonstandard treatments have not been tested and proven to be effective for treating cancer.

As you consider your options, here are 3 important steps you can take:

- Talk to your doctor or nurse about any treatment you are thinking about using.
- Check the list of "red flags," below.
- Contact the American Cancer Society at **800-227-2345** to learn more about complementary and alternative treatments in general and to learn more about the specific treatments you are considering.

Red flags

You can use the questions below to spot treatments or methods to avoid. A "yes" answer to any one of these questions should raise a red flag.

- Does the treatment promise a cure?
- Are you told not to use standard medical treatment?
- Is the treatment or drug a "secret" that only certain people can give?
- Does the treatment require you to travel to another country?
- Do the promoters attack the medical or scientific community?

The decision is yours

Decisions about how to treat or manage your cancer are always yours to make. If you are thinking about using a complementary or alternative method, be sure to learn about it and talk with your doctor about it. With reliable information and the support of your health care team, you may be able to safely use methods that can help you while avoiding those that could be harmful.

Considering Prostate Cancer Treatment Options

If you have prostate cancer, there are many important factors to take into account before deciding on a treatment option, such as your age and general health and the likelihood that the cancer will cause problems for you. You should also think about which side effects you can live with. Some men, for example, cannot imagine living with side effects such as incontinence or impotence. Other men are less concerned about these side effects and more concerned about removing or destroying the cancer.

If you are older or have other serious health problems and your cancer is slow growing, you might find it helpful to think of prostate cancer as a chronic disease that will probably not lead to your death but may cause symptoms you want to avoid. You may be more inclined to consider active surveillance (careful follow-up with your doctor) or hormone therapy and less inclined to consider treatments that are likely to cause major side effects, such as radiation and surgery. Of course, age itself is not necessarily the best basis on which to make your choice. Many men are in good mental and physical shape at age 70, while some younger men may not be as healthy.

If you are younger and otherwise healthy, you might be more willing to put up with the side effects of treatment if they offer you the best chance for cure. Most doctors now believe that external radiation, radical prostatectomy, and brachytherapy (radioactive implants) have about the same cure rates for the earliest-stage prostate cancers. However, there are pros and cons to each type of treatment that should be considered, including possible risks and side effects (described earlier in this chapter).

This issue is complicated even further by the explosion of newer types of surgery (laparoscopic prostatectomy and robotic-assisted prostatectomy) and radiation therapy (conformal radiation therapy, intensity-modulated radiation therapy, proton beam radiation, etc.) in recent years. Many of these appear very promising, but there is very little long-term data on them, which means comparing them to each other is very difficult, if not impossible.

Such a complex decision is often hard to make by yourself. You may find it helpful to talk with your family and friends before making a decision. Prostate cancer is not a uniform disease, and each man's experience with it is different. Just because someone you know had a good (or bad) experience with a certain type of treatment doesn't necessarily mean the same will be true for you.

You may also want to consider getting more than one medical opinion, perhaps even from different types of doctors. For early-stage cancers, it is natural for surgical specialists, such as urologists, to favor surgery and for radiation oncologists to lean more toward radiation. Doctors specializing in newer types of treatment may be more likely to recommend their therapies. Talking to each of them may give you a better perspective on your options. Your primary care doctor may also be helpful in sorting out which treatment might be right for you.

You might find that speaking with others who have faced or are currently facing the same issues is useful. The American Cancer Society's program, Man to Man, and similar programs sponsored by other organizations provide a forum for you to meet and discuss these and other cancer-related issues. For more information about available programs, contact your American Cancer Society toll-free at **800-227-2345** or on the Web at **cancer.org**.

Before Deciding on Treatment

The information in the following sections describes the main treatment options available for prostate cancer in different situations. Before deciding on treatment, here are some further questions you may want to ask yourself:

- Are you the type of person who needs to do something about your cancer, even if it might result in serious side effects? Or would you be comfortable with active surveillance, even if it means you might have more anxiety (and need more frequent follow-up) in the future?
- Do you feel the need to know right away whether your doctor thinks he or she was able to get all of the cancer out (a reason some men choose surgery)? Or are you comfortable with not knowing the results of treatment for a while (as is the case in radiation therapy) if it means not having to have surgery?
- Do you prefer to go with the newest technology, which may have some

theoretical advantages? Or do you prefer to go with treatment methods that are better proven and with which doctors may have more experience?

- Which potential treatment side effects (incontinence, impotence, bowel problems) might be most distressing to you?
- How important for you are issues like the amount of time spent in treatment or recovery?
- If your initial treatment is not successful, what would your options be at that point?

Many men find it very stressful to have to choose between treatment options and are very fearful they will choose the "wrong" one. In many cases, there is no single best option. It's important to take your time and decide which option is right for you.

Initial Treatment of Prostate Cancer by Stage

The "How Is Prostate Cancer Staged?" section of this document explains how the T, N, and M classifications are used to stage your cancer. The stage of your cancer is one of the most important factors in choosing the best way to treat it.

What follows is a description of the treatments that may be options for men with prostate cancer diagnosed at a specific stage. But keep in mind that other factors, such as age, life expectancy, and risk of cancer recurrence after treatment (based on factors like Gleason score and PSA level) must also be taken into account when looking at treatment options.

Stage I: T1a, N0, M0, with a low Gleason score (2 to 4)

These prostate cancers are small (T1 or T2a) and have not grown outside of the prostate. They have low Gleason scores (6 or less) and low PSA levels (less than 10). They usually grow very slowly and may never cause any symptoms or other health problems.

For men without any prostate cancer symptoms who are elderly and/or have other serious health problems, active surveillance is often recommended. For men who wish to start treatment, radiation therapy (external beam or brachytherapy) or androgen deprivation may be options.

Men who are younger and healthy may consider active surveillance, radical prostatectomy, or radiation therapy (external beam or brachytherapy).

Stage II

Stage II cancers have not yet grown outside of the prostate gland, but are larger (T2), have higher Gleason scores and/or higher PSA levels than stage I tumors. Compared with stage I prostate cancers, stage II cancers that are not treated with surgery or radiation are more likely to eventually spread beyond the prostate and cause symptoms.

As with stage I cancers, active surveillance by following PSA levels is often a good option for men whose cancer is not causing any symptoms and who are elderly and/or have other serious health problems. Radical prostatectomy and radiation therapy (external beam or brachytherapy) may also be appropriate options.

Treatment options for men who are younger and otherwise healthy may include the following:

- radical prostatectomy (often with removal of the **pelvic lymph nodes**). This procedure may be followed by external beam radiation if your cancer is found to have spread beyond the prostate at the time of surgery, or if the PSA level is still detectable several weeks after surgery.
- external beam radiation only*
- brachytherapy only*
- brachytherapy and external beam radiation combined*
- taking part in a clinical trial of newer treatments

Stage III

Stage III cancers have grown outside of the prostate capsule but have not reached the bladder or rectum (T3). They have not spread to lymph nodes (N0) or distant organs (M0). These cancers are more likely to come back (recur) after treatment than earlier stage tumors.

Treatment options at this stage may include the following:

- external beam radiation plus hormone therapy
- hormone therapy only
- radical prostatectomy in selected cases (often with removal of the pelvic lymph

---

*All the radiation options may be combined with several months of hormone therapy if there is a greater chance of recurrence based on PSA level and/or Gleason score.

nodes). This may be followed by radiation therapy.

- active surveillance for those who have another more serious illness
- taking part in a clinical trial of newer treatments

Stage IV

Stage IV cancers have already spread to the bladder or rectum (T4), lymph nodes (N1), or distant organs such as the bones (M1). These cancers are generally not considered to be curable.

Treatment options may include the following:

- hormone therapy
- external beam radiation plus hormone therapy (in selected cases)
- surgery (TURP) to relieve symptoms such as bleeding or urinary obstruction
- active surveillance for those who have another serious illness
- taking part in a clinical trial of newer treatments

If symptoms are not relieved by standard treatments and the cancer continues to grow and spread, chemotherapy may be an option. You may also want to think about taking part in a clinical trial. Treatment of stage IV prostate cancer may also include treatments for relief of symptoms such as bone pain.

Following PSA Levels After Treatment Meant to Cure Prostate Cancer

The PSA level is often a good indicator of whether or not initial treatment was successful. Generally speaking, your PSA level should get very low after treatment. But PSA results are not always clear-cut, and sometimes doctors aren't sure what they mean.

After surgery

The PSA should fall to an undetectable level within a couple of months after radical prostatectomy. Because some PSA may remain in the blood for several weeks after surgery, even if all of the prostate cells were removed, doctors often advise waiting at least 6 to 8 weeks after surgery before getting the test.

Blood tests have become much more sensitive in recent years—so sensitive that they can detect very small amounts of PSA. This development would seem to be a good thing, but it has made it more difficult to define exactly what an "undetectable" PSA level is. For example, a PSA of 0.5 (ng/mL) after surgery might be concerning, but doctors are not certain whether levels of 0.01 or 0.02 should cause concern. Some doctors would advise following such PSA levels over time to get a better idea of what may be going on, possibly with repeat tests every few months. Others might be more inclined to recommend further treatment. Of course, this uncertainty can be very stressful for patients and their families.

After radiation therapy

The different types of radiation therapy don't kill all of the cells in the prostate gland, so they are not expected to cause the PSA to drop to an undetectable level. The remaining normal prostate cells will continue to make some PSA.

The pattern of the drop in PSA after radiation is also different than that shown with surgery. PSA levels after radiation tend to drop gradually and may not reach their lowest level until 2 years or more after treatment.

Doctors tend to follow the PSA levels every few months to look for trends. A one-time, small rise in PSA might be a cause for closer monitoring, but it may not necessarily mean that the cancer has returned, as PSA levels may fluctuate slightly from time to time. However, a PSA that is rising on consecutive tests after treatment might indicate that cancer is still present. Some medical groups have proposed that a PSA rise of more than 2 above the lowest level the PSA has reached should be used as the cutoff point, but not all doctors agree with this recommendation.

There is also a phenomenon called a "PSA bounce" that sometimes happens after radiation therapy. The PSA rises slightly for a short time within the first couple of years after treatment, but then falls back down. Doctors aren't sure why this happens, but it does not appear to affect the patient's prognosis.

Prostate Cancer that Remains or Recurs After Treatment

If the PSA level shows that the prostate cancer has not been cured or has come back (recurred) after an initial attempt to cure it, further treatment may be an option. Follow-up therapy will depend on where the cancer is thought to be located and what treatment(s) you have already had. Usually, the same type of treatment is not an option because of the increased potential for serious side effects. For example, men who have already had radiation therapy to the prostate cannot have that area treated with radiation again. Imaging tests such as CT, MRI, or bone scans may be done to get a better idea about where the cancer may be.

If the cancer is still thought to be localized to the area of the prostate, a second attempt at **curative treatment** may be possible. If you've had a radical prostatectomy, radiation therapy may be an option. If your first treatment was radiation, treatment options include cryosurgery or radical prostatectomy, but when radical prostatectomy is done after radiation, it does carry a higher risk for potential side effects.

If the cancer has spread outside the prostate gland, it will most likely go first to nearby lymph nodes, and then to the bones. Much less often the cancer will spread to the liver or other organs.

When prostate cancer has spread to other parts of the body (including the bones), hormone therapy is probably the most effective treatment, but it is very unlikely to cure the cancer. Usually, the first treatment is an LHRH analog. If this stops working, an antiandrogen may be added. Other hormonal agents such as ketoconazole or estrogens (female hormones) may be helpful and can sometimes slow or stop the cancer from growing. Hormone therapy will be given as long as the cancer is responding (based on the PSA level and whether or not symptoms develop).

Remember that prostate cancer is usually slow growing, so even if it does come back, it may not cause problems for many years. In a Johns Hopkins University study of men whose PSA level began to rise after surgery, there was an average of about 8 years before there were **signs** the cancer had spread to distant parts of the body. Of course, these signs appeared earlier in some men and later in others.

Hormone-refractory prostate cancer (HRPC)

Cancer that no longer responds to hormone therapy such as LHRH analogs or antiandrogens is considered hormone-refractory, and can be hard to treat. At one time, it was thought that chemotherapy was not effective against prostate cancer, but in recent years this notion has been challenged. Several chemotherapy drugs have been shown to reduce PSA levels and improve quality of life. Recent studies of chemotherapy regimens that include the drug docetaxel (Taxotere) have shown that it can improve survival by an average of several months, as well as reduce cancer pain. The cancer vaccine sipuleucel-T (Provenge) may also help prolong life for men with prostate cancer that no longer responds to hormone therapy.

Bisphosphonates appear to be helpful for many men whose cancer has spread to the bones. These drugs can reduce pain and even slow cancer growth in many cases. There are also other medicines and methods to keep pain and other symptoms under control. External radiation therapy can help treat bone pain if it is only in a few spots. Radioactive strontium or samarium may reduce pain if it is more widespread and may also slow the growth of the cancer.

If you are having pain from your prostate cancer, make sure your doctor is aware of this condition. There are many very effective drugs that can relieve pain. But for relief to happen, you must make it clear to your doctor that you have pain. For more information about managing cancer pain, contact your American Cancer Society at **800-227-2345** or on the Web at **cancer.org** and request the document *Advanced Cancer*.

There are several promising new agents now being tested against prostate cancer, including vaccines, monoclonal antibodies, and differentiating agents. Because the ability to treat hormone-refractory prostate cancer is still not good enough, men are encouraged to explore new options by taking part in clinical trials.

Your Medical Team

Your cancer care team comprises several people, each with a different type of expertise to contribute to your care. One of your team members will take the lead in coordinating your care. Most prostate cancer patients choose a medical oncologist or urologist to lead the team. It should be clear to all team members who is in charge, and that person should inform the others of your progress.

This alphabetical list will acquaint you with the health care professionals you may encounter, depending on which treatment option and follow-up path you choose, and their areas of expertise:

Anesthesiologist

An anesthesiologist is a medical doctor who administers anesthesia (drugs or gases) to make you sleep and be unconscious or to prevent or relieve pain during and after a surgical procedure.

Dietitian

A dietitian is specially trained to help you make healthy diet choices and maintain a healthy weight before, during, and after treatment. Dietitians can help patients deal with side effects of treatment, such as nausea, vomiting, or sore throat. A registered dietitian (RD) has at least a bachelor's degree and has passed a national competency examination.

Genetic counselor

A genetic counselor is a health professional trained to help people through the process of genetic testing. A genetic counselor can explain the available tests to you, discuss the pros and cons, and address any concerns you might have. This counselor can arrange for genetic testing and then help interpret the test results. A certified genetic counselor has at least a master's degree and has passed both a general competency examination and a specialty genetic counseling examination.

Medical oncologist

A medical oncologist (also sometimes called an oncologist) is a medical doctor you may see after diagnosis. The oncologist is a cancer expert who understands specific types of cancer, their treatments, and their causes. He or she may help cancer patients make decisions about a course of treatment and then manage all phases of cancer care. Oncologists most often become involved when you need chemotherapy, but can also prescribe hormonal therapy and other anticancer drugs.

Nurses

During your treatment you will be in contact with different types of nurses.

Clinical nurse specialist: A clinical nurse specialist (CNS) is a nurse who has a master's degree in a specific area, such as oncology, psychiatry, or critical care nursing. The CNS often provides expertise to staff and may provide special services to patients, such as leading support groups and coordinating cancer care.

Nurse practitioner: A nurse practitioner is a registered nurse with a master's degree or doctoral degree who can manage the care of patients with prostate cancer and has additional training in primary care. He or she shares many tasks with your doctors, such as recording your medical history, conducting physical examinations, and doing follow-up care. In most states, a nurse practitioner can prescribe medications with a doctor's supervision.

Oncology-certified nurse: An oncology-certified nurse is a clinical nurse who has demonstrated an in-depth knowledge of oncology care. He or she has passed a certification examination. Oncology-certified nurses are found in all areas of cancer practice.

Registered nurse: A registered nurse has an associate or bachelor's degree in nursing and has passed a state licensing examination. He or she can monitor your condition, provide treatment, educate you about side effects, and help you adjust to cancer, both physically and emotionally.

Pain specialist

Pain specialists are doctors, nurses, and pharmacists who are experts in managing pain. They can help you find pain control methods that are effective and allow you to maintain your quality of life. Not all doctors and nurses are trained in pain care, so you may have to request a pain specialist if your pain relief needs are not being met.

Pathologist

A pathologist is a medical doctor specially trained in diagnosing disease based on examination of microscopic tissue and fluid samples. He or she will determine the classification (cell type) of your cancer, help determine the stage (extent) and grade (estimate of aggressiveness) of your cancer, and issue a pathology report so that you and your doctor can decide on treatment options.

Personal or primary care physician

A personal physician may be a general doctor, internist, or family practice doctor. He or she is often the medical doctor you first saw when you noticed symptoms of illness. This general or family practice doctor may be a member of your medical team, but a specialist is most often a patient's cancer care team leader.

Physician assistant

Physicians assistants (PAs) are health care professionals licensed to practice medicine with physician supervision. Physician assistants practice in the areas of primary care medicine (family medicine, internal medicine, pediatrics, and obstetrics and gynecology), as well as in surgery and the surgical subspecialties. Under the supervision of a doctor, they can diagnose and treat medical problems and, in most states, can also prescribe medications.

Psychologist or psychiatrist

A psychologist is a licensed mental health professional who is often part of the cancer care team. He or she provides counseling on emotional and psychological issues. A psychologist may have specialized training and experience in treating people with cancer.

A psychiatrist is a medical doctor specializing in mental health and behavioral disorders. Psychiatrists provide counseling and can also prescribe medications.

Radiation oncologist

A radiation oncologist is a medical doctor who specializes in treating cancer by using therapeutic radiation (high-energy x-rays or seeds). If you choose radiation, the radiation oncologist evaluates you frequently during the course of treatment and at intervals afterward. The radiation oncologist will usually work closely with your oncologist and will help you make decisions about radiation therapy options. A radiation oncologist is assisted by a radiation therapist during treatment and works with a radiation physicist, an expert who is trained in ensuring that you receive the correct dose of radiation treatment. The physicist is also assisted by a dosimetrist, a technician who helps plan and calculate the dosage, number, and length of your radiation treatments.

Radiation physicist: A radiation physicist ensures that the radiation machine delivers the right amount of radiation to the correct site in the body. The physicist works with the radiation oncologist to choose the treatment schedule and dose that will have the best chance of killing the most cancer cells.

Radiologist

A radiologist is a medical doctor specializing in the use of imaging procedures (for example, diagnostic x-rays, ultrasound, magnetic resonance images, and bone scans) that produce pictures of internal body structures. He or she has special training in diagnosing cancer and other diseases and interpreting the results of imaging procedures. Your radiologist issues a radiology report describing the findings to your urologist or radiation oncologist. The radiology images and report may be used to aid in diagnosis; to help classify and determine the extent of your illness; to help locate tumors during procedures, surgery, and radiation

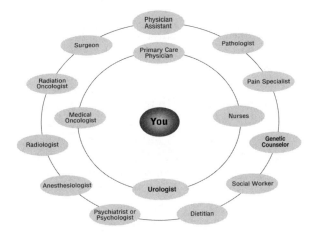

treatment; or to look for the possible spread or recurrence of the cancer after treatment.

Social worker

A social worker is a health specialist, usually with a master's degree, who is licensed or certified by the state in which he or she works. A social worker is an expert in coordinating and providing social services. He or she is trained to help you and your family deal with a range of emotional and practical challenges, such as finances, child care, emotional issues, family concerns and relationships, transportation, and problems with the health care system. If your social worker is trained in cancer-related problems, he or she can counsel you about your fears or concerns, help answer questions about diagnosis and treatment, and lead cancer support groups. You may communicate with your social worker during a hospital stay or on an outpatient basis.

Surgeon

Different types of surgeons provide treatment for prostate cancer. A general surgeon is trained to operate on all parts of the body, including the prostate. A surgical urologist is a surgeon who has had advanced training in the surgical treatment of people with prostate cancer. Cancer centers usually have one or more such individuals on their staff. If you require surgery as part of your treatment, the surgeon will perform the operation and then manage any side effects you might have. He or she will also issue a report to your other doctors to help determine the rest of your treatment plan.

Urologist

A urologist is a medical doctor who specializes in diagnosis and treatment of the urinary tract in men and women and of the genital area in men.

More Treatment Information

For more details on treatment options—including some that may not be addressed in this book—the National Comprehensive Cancer Network (NCCN) and the National Cancer Institute (NCI) are good sources of information.

The NCCN, made up of experts from many of the nation's leading cancer centers, develops cancer treatment guidelines for doctors. These are available on the NCCN Web site (**www.nccn.org**).

The NCI provides treatment guidelines via its telephone information center (**800-4-CANCER**) and its Web site (**www.cancer.gov**). Detailed guidelines intended for use by cancer care professionals are also available on **www.cancer.gov**.

Questions
to Ask

What Should You Ask Your Doctor About Prostate Cancer?

It is important for you to have honest, open discussions with your cancer care team. They want to answer all of your questions, no matter how minor you might think they are. Consider these questions:

- What are the chances that the cancer has spread beyond my prostate? If so, is it still curable?
- What further tests (if any) do you recommend, and why?
- What is the clinical stage and Gleason score (grade) of my cancer? What do those mean in my case?
- What is my expected survival rate based on clinical stage, grade, and various treatment options?
- Should I consider active surveillance as an option? Why or why not?
- Do you recommend a radical prostatectomy or radiation? Why or why not?

- If you recommend radical prostatectomy, will it be nerve sparing?
- Should I consider laparoscopic or robot-assisted prostatectomy?
- What types of radiation therapy might work best for me?
- What other treatment(s) might be right for me? Why?
- Among those treatments, what are the risks or side effects that I should expect?
- What are the chances that I will have problems with incontinence or impotence?
- What are the chances that I will have other urinary or rectal problems?
- What are the chances of recurrence of my cancer with the treatment programs we have discussed? What would be our next step if this happened?
- Should I follow a special diet?

In addition to these sample questions, be sure to write down some of your own. For instance, you might want to ask about recovery time so that you can plan your work schedule. If you are younger, you may want to discuss your plans for children if there is a possibility you could become impotent or sterile. You also may want to ask about second opinions or about clinical trials for which you may qualify.

After Treatment

What Happens After Treatment for Prostate Cancer?

Completing treatment can be both stressful and exciting. You will be relieved to finish treatment, yet it is hard not to worry about cancer coming back. (When cancer returns, it is called recurrence.) This is a very common concern among those who have had cancer.

It may take a while before your confidence in your own recovery begins to feel real and your fears are somewhat relieved. To learn more about what to look for and how to learn to live with the possibility of cancer coming back, contact your American Cancer Society at **800-227-2345** or on the Web at **cancer.org** and request the document *Living With Uncertainty: The Fear of Cancer Recurrence*.

Follow-up Care

After treatment for prostate cancer, your doctor will want to watch you carefully, checking to see if your cancer recurs or spreads further. Your doctor should also outline a follow-up plan. This plan usually includes regular doctor visits, prostate-specific antigen (PSA) blood tests, and digital rectal exams (DREs), which will likely begin within a few months of finishing treatment. Most doctors recommend PSA tests about every 6 months for the first 5 years after treatment, and at least yearly after that. Bone scans or other imaging tests may also be done, depending on your medical situation. This is the time for you to ask your health care team any questions you need answered and to discuss any concerns you might have.

Almost any cancer treatment can have side effects. Some may last for a few weeks to several months, but others can be permanent. Don't hesitate to tell your cancer care team about any symptoms or side effects that bother you so they can help you manage them.

It is also important to keep medical insurance. Even though no one wants to think of his cancer coming back, it is always a possibility. If it happens, you should not have to worry about paying for treatment. Should your cancer come back, you can learn more about how to manage and cope with this phase of treatment by calling your American Cancer Society at **800-227-2345** or on the Web at **cancer.org** to request the document *When Your Cancer Comes Back: Cancer Recurrence.*

Prostate cancer can recur many years after initial treatment, which is why it is important to keep regular doctor visits and report any new symptoms (such as bone pain or problems with urination). Should your prostate cancer come back, your treatment options will depend on where it is thought to be located and what types of treatment you have already had. For more information, see the section, "How is Prostate Cancer Treated?"

Seeing a New Doctor

At some point after your cancer diagnosis and treatment, you may find yourself in the office of a new doctor. Your original doctor may have moved or retired, or you may have moved or changed doctors for some reason. It is important that you be able to give your new doctor the exact details of your cancer diagnosis and treatment. Make sure you have the following information handy:

- a copy of your pathology report from any biopsy or surgery
- if you had surgery, a copy of your operative report
- if you had radiation therapy, a copy of your treatment summary
- if you were hospitalized, a copy of the discharge summary that every doctor must prepare when patients are sent home from the hospital
- finally, since some drugs can have long-term side effects, a list of your drugs, drug doses, and when you took them

Lifestyle Changes to Consider During and After Treatment

Having cancer and dealing with treatment can be time-consuming and emotionally draining, but it can also be a time to look at your life in new ways.

Maybe you are thinking about how to improve your health over the long term. Some people even begin this process during cancer treatment.

Make healthier choices

Think about your life before you learned you had cancer. Were there things you did that might have made you less healthy? Maybe you drank too much alcohol, or ate more than you needed, or smoked, or didn't exercise very often. Emotionally, maybe you kept your feelings bottled up, or maybe you let stressful situations go on too long.

Now is not the time to feel guilty or to blame yourself. However, you can start making changes *today* that can have positive effects for the rest of your life. Not only will you feel better but you will also be healthier. What better time than now to take advantage of the motivation you have as a result of going through a life-changing experience like having cancer?

You can start by working on those things that you feel most concerned about. Get help with those that are harder for you. For instance, if you are thinking about quitting smoking and need help, call the American Cancer Society at **800-227-2345** for information about smoking cessation programs.

Diet and nutrition

Eating right can be a challenge for anyone, but it can get even tougher during and after cancer treatment. For instance, treatment often may change your sense of taste. Nausea can be a problem. You may lose your appetite for a while and lose weight when you don't want to. On the other hand, some people gain weight even without eating more. This can be frustrating, too.

If you are losing weight or have taste problems during treatment, do the best you can with eating and remember that these problems usually improve over time. You may want to ask your cancer care team for a referral to a dietitian, an expert in nutrition who can give you ideas on how to fight some of the side effects of your treatment. You may also find it helps to eat small portions every 2 to 3 hours until you feel better and can go back to a more normal schedule.

One of the best things you can do after treatment is to put healthy eating habits into place. You will be surprised at the long-term benefits of some simple changes, like increasing the variety of healthy foods you eat. Try to eat 5 or more servings of vegetables and fruits each day. Choose whole grain foods instead of white flour and sugars. Try to limit meats that are high in fat. Cut back on processed meats like hot dogs, bologna, and bacon. Get rid of them altogether if you can. If you drink alcohol, limit yourself to 1 or 2 drinks a day at the most. And don't forget to get some type of regular exercise. The combination of a good diet and regular exercise will help you maintain a healthy weight and keep you feeling more energetic.

Rest, fatigue, work, and exercise

Fatigue is a very common symptom in people being treated for cancer. This side effect is often not an ordinary type of tiredness but a "bone-weary" exhaustion that doesn't get better with rest. For some, this fatigue lasts a long time after treatment and can discourage them from physical activity.

However, exercise can actually help you reduce fatigue. Studies have shown that patients who follow an exercise program tailored to their personal needs feel physically and emotionally better and can more effectively cope.

If you are ill and need to be on bed rest during treatment, it is normal to expect your fitness, endurance, and muscle strength to decline some. Physical therapy can help you maintain strength and range of motion in your muscles, which can help fight fatigue and the sense of depression that sometimes comes with feeling so tired.

Any program of physical activity should fit your own situation. An older person who has never exercised will not be able to take on the same amount of exercise as a 20-year-old who plays tennis 3 times a week. If you haven't exercised in a few years but can still get around, you may want to think about taking short walks.

Talk with your health care team before starting, and get their opinion about your exercise plans. Then, try to get an exercise buddy so that you're not doing it alone. Having family or friends involved when starting a new exercise program can give you that extra boost of support to keep you going when the push just isn't there.

If you are very tired, though, you will need to balance activity with rest. It is okay to rest when you need to. It is really hard for some people to allow themselves to do that when they are used to working all day or taking care of a household.

For more information about fatigue, please contact your American Cancer Society at **800-227-2345** or on the Web at **cancer.org** and request the documents *Fatigue in People with Cancer* and *Anemia in People with Cancer.*

Exercise can improve your physical and emotional health in the following ways:

- It improves your cardiovascular (heart and circulation) fitness.
- It strengthens your muscles.
- It reduces fatigue.
- It lowers anxiety and depression.
- It makes you feel generally happier.
- It helps you feel better about yourself.

And long term, we know that exercise plays a role in preventing some cancers. The American Cancer Society, in its guidelines on physical activity for cancer prevention, recommends that adults take part in at least 30 minutes of moderate to vigorous physical activity, above usual activities, on 5 or more days of the week; 45 to 60 minutes of intentional physical activity is preferable.

How About Your Emotional Health?

Once your treatment ends, you may find yourself overwhelmed by emotions. This reaction happens to a lot of people. You may have been going through so much during treatment that you could only focus on getting through your treatment.

Now you may find that you think about the potential of your own death or the effect of your cancer on your family, friends, and career. You may also begin to re-evaluate your relationship with your spouse or partner. Unexpected issues may also cause concern—for instance, as you become healthier and have fewer doctor visits, you will see your health care team less often. That can be a source of anxiety for some.

This is an ideal time to seek out emotional and social support. You need people you can turn to for strength and comfort. Support can come in many forms: family, friends, cancer support groups, church or spiritual groups, online support communities, or individual counselors.

Almost everyone who has been through cancer can benefit from getting some type of support. What's best for you depends on your situation and personality. Some people feel safe in peer-support groups or education groups. Others would rather talk in an informal setting, such as church. Others may feel more at ease talking one-on-one with a trusted friend or counselor. Whatever your source of strength or comfort, make sure you have a place to go with your concerns.

The cancer journey can feel very lonely. It is not necessary or realistic to go it all by yourself. And your friends and family may feel shut out if you decide not include them. Let them in—and let in anyone else who you feel may help. If you aren't sure who can help, call your American Cancer Society at **800-227-2345** to learn about appropriate groups and resources in your area.

You can't change the fact that you have had cancer. What you can change is how you live the rest of your life—making healthful choices and feeling as well as possible, physically and emotionally.

What Happens If Treatment Is No Longer Working?

If cancer continues to grow after one kind of treatment, or if it returns, it is often possible to try another treatment plan that might still cure the cancer, or at least shrink the tumors enough to help you live longer and feel better. On the other hand, when a person has received several different medical treatments and the cancer has not been cured, over time the cancer tends to become resistant to all treatment. At this time it's important to weigh the possible limited benefit of a new treatment against the possible downsides, including continued doctor visits and treatment side effects.

Everyone has his or her own way of looking at this situation. Some people may want to focus on remaining comfortable during their limited time left.

This is likely to be the most difficult time in your battle with cancer—when you have tried everything medically within reason and it's just not working anymore. Although your doctor may offer you new treatment, you need to consider that, at some point, continuing treatment is not likely to improve your health or change your prognosis or survival.

If you want to continue treatment to fight your cancer as long as you can, you still need to consider the odds of more treatment having any benefit. In many cases, your doctor can estimate the response rate for the treatment you are considering. Some people are tempted to try more chemotherapy or radiation, for example, even when their doctors say that the odds of benefit are less than 1%. In this situation, you need to think about and understand your reasons for choosing this plan.

No matter what you decide to do, it is important that you be as comfortable as possible. Make sure you are asking for and getting treatment for any symptoms you might have, such as pain. This type of treatment is called **palliative treatment**.

Palliative treatment helps relieve symptoms, but is not expected to cure the disease; its main purpose is to improve your quality of life. Sometimes, the treatments you get to control your symptoms are similar to the treatments used to treat cancer. For example, radiation therapy might be given to help relieve bone pain from bone metastasis. Or chemotherapy might be given to help shrink a tumor and keep it from causing a bowel obstruction. But this is not the same as receiving treatment to try to cure the cancer.

At some point, you may benefit from **hospice** care. Most of the time, this care is given at home. Your cancer may be causing symptoms or problems that need attention, and hospice focuses on your comfort. You should know that receiving hospice care doesn't mean you can't have treatment for the problems caused by your cancer or other health conditions. It just means that the focus of your care is on living life as fully as possible and feeling as well as you can at this difficult stage of your cancer.

Remember also that maintaining hope is important. Your hope for a cure may not be as bright, but there is still hope for good times with family and friends—times that are filled with happiness and meaning. In a way, pausing at this time in your cancer treatment is an opportunity to refocus on the most important things in your life. This is the time to do some things you've always wanted to do and to stop doing the things you no longer want to do.

Latest Research

What's New in Prostate Cancer Research and Treatment?

Research into the causes, prevention, and treatment of prostate cancer is under way in many medical centers throughout the world.

Genetics

New research on genes linked to prostate cancer is helping scientists better understand how prostate cancer develops. These studies are expected to provide answers about the genetic changes that lead to prostate cancer. This research could make it possible to design medicines to reverse those changes. Tests to find abnormal prostate cancer genes could also help identify men at high risk who would benefit from more intensive screening or from chemoprevention trials, which use drugs to try to keep them from getting cancer.

Most of the genes that have been studied so far are from chromosomes that are inherited from both parents. One recent study found that a certain variant of mitochondrial DNA, which is inherited only from a person's mother, might double or even triple a man's risk for prostate cancer.

An exciting new development in genetics research is the use of DNA microarray technology, which allows scientists to study thousands of genes at the same time. Using this method, researchers have identified several genes now thought to play a role in prostate cancer. This research may eventually provide a more sensitive screening test for prostate cancer than the PSA blood test currently in use.

One of the biggest problems now facing men with prostate cancer and their doctors is determining which cancers are likely to stay within the gland and which ones are more likely to grow and spread (and definitely need treatment). New discoveries may help with this some time in the near future. For example, the product of one gene identified by DNA microarray, known as EZH2, seems to appear more often in advanced prostate cancers than in those at an early stage. Researchers are now trying to decide whether the presence of this gene product, or others, indicates that a cancer is more aggressive. This information could eventually help tell which men need treatment and which men might be better served by watchful waiting.

Prevention

Researchers continue to look for foods that increase or decrease prostate cancer risk. Scientists have found some substances in tomatoes (lycopenes) and soybeans (isoflavones) that may help prevent prostate cancer. Studies are now looking at the possible effects of these compounds more closely. Scientists are also trying to develop related compounds that are even more potent and might be used as dietary supplements. So far, most research suggests that a balanced diet including these foods as well as other fruits and vegetables is of greater benefit than taking these substances as dietary supplements.

Some studies have suggested that certain vitamin and mineral supplements (such as vitamin E and selenium) might lower prostate cancer risk. But a large study of this issue, called the Selenium and Vitamin E Cancer Prevention Trial (SELECT), found that neither vitamin E nor selenium supplements lowered prostate cancer risk after daily use for about 5 years.

Vitamin D is another vitamin that may be important to prostate cancer risk. Recent studies have found that men with high levels of vitamin D seem to have a lower risk for the more lethal forms of prostate cancer to develop. Overall, though, studies have not found that Vitamin D is protective for prostate cancer.

Many people assume that vitamins are natural substances that cause no harm, but recent research has shown that high doses may be harmful. One study found that men who take more than 7 multivitamin tablets per week may have an increased risk for advanced prostate cancer.

Scientists are also testing certain hormonal medicines as a way of reducing prostate cancer risk. Finasteride (Proscar) and dutasteride (Avodart) are drugs that lower the body's levels of a potent androgen called DHT. Both drugs are already used to treat benign prostatic hyperplasia (BPH). The results of one such study, the Prostate Cancer Prevention Trial are discussed in the section "Can Prostate Cancer Be Prevented?" This study looked at the possible benefits of finasteride, although the results were not clear-cut. Another study is looking at whether dutasteride might be helpful in reducing the risk of prostate cancer.

Early Detection

Doctors agree that the PSA blood test is not a perfect test for finding prostate cancer early. It misses some cancers and, in other cases, it is elevated when cancer isn't present. Researchers are working on 2 strategies to address this problem.

One approach is to try to improve on the test that measures the total PSA level, as described in the section "Can Prostate Cancer Be Found Early?" The percent-free PSA may be considered an improvement over the PSA test; however, the percent-free PSA requires 2 separate tests. Another option might be to measure only the complexed PSA (the portion of PSA that is not free) to begin with, instead of the total and free PSA. This one test could give the same amount of information as the other 2 done separately. Studies are now under way to see if this test provides the same level of accuracy.

The other approach is to develop new tests based on other **tumor markers**. Several newer blood tests seem to be more accurate than the PSA test, based on early studies. Another approach is to look for signs of the body's own immune reaction to substances made by prostate cancer cells. While early results have been promising, these and other new tests are not yet available outside of research laboratories and will require more study before they are widely used to test for prostate cancer.

Other new tests under study are urine tests. One test looks at the level of something called prostate cancer gene 3 (PCA3) in the urine. The higher the level, the more likely that prostate cancer is present. In studies, it was used along with the PSA test. Another test looks for an abnormal gene called TMPRSS2:ERG in prostate cells. The cells to be tested are found in urine given after a rectal exam. This gene is found in about half of all localized prostate cancers. It is rarely found in the cells of men without prostate cancer. Studies are under way to develop this into a test for early detection of prostate cancer.

Diagnosis

Doctors performing prostate biopsies often rely on transrectal ultrasound (TRUS), which creates black and white images of the prostate by using sound waves, to know where to take samples from. But standard ultrasound may not detect some areas containing cancer. A newer approach is to measure blood flow within the gland by using a technique called color Doppler ultrasound. (Tumors often have more blood vessels around them than normal tissue.) It may make prostate biopsies more accurate by helping to ensure that the right part of the gland is sampled. An even newer technique may further enhance color Doppler. It involves first injecting the patient with a contrast material containing microbubbles. Promising results have been reported, but more studies will be needed before its use becomes common.

Staging

Staging plays a key role in determining a man's treatment options. But imaging tests for prostate cancer such as CT and MRI scans cannot detect all cancers, especially small areas of cancer in lymph nodes. A newer method, called enhanced MRI, may help find lymph nodes that contain cancer. Patients first have a standard MRI. They are then injected with tiny magnetic particles and have another scan done the next day. Differences between the 2 scans point to possible cancer cells in the lymph nodes. Early results of this technique are promising, but it needs more research before it becomes widely used.

Treatment

Treatment is a very active area of research. Newer treatments are being developed, and improvements are being made among many standard prostate cancer treatment methods.

Surgery

If the nerves that control erections (which run along either side of the prostate) must be removed during the operation, a man will become impotent. Some doctors are now exploring the use of nerve grafts to replace cut nerves and restore potency.

These grafts could be nerves removed from other parts of the body, or they might be something artificial. This technique is still considered experimental, and not all doctors agree as to its usefulness. Further study is under way.

Radiation therapy

As described in the section, "How Is Prostate Cancer Treated?" advances in technology are making it possible to aim radiation more precisely than in the past. Currently used methods such as conformal radiation therapy (CRT), intensity modulated radiation therapy (IMRT), and proton beam radiation allow doctors to treat only the prostate gland and avoid radiation to normal tissues as much as possible. These methods are expected to increase the effectiveness of radiation therapy while reducing the side effects. Studies are being done to find out which radiation techniques are best suited for specific groups of patients with prostate cancer.

Technology is making other forms of radiation therapy more effective as well. New computer programs allow doctors to better plan the radiation doses and approaches for both external radiation therapy and brachytherapy. Planning for brachytherapy can now even be done during the procedure (intraoperatively).

Newer treatments for localized disease

Researchers are looking at newer forms of treatment for early-stage prostate cancer. These new treatments could be used either as the first type of treatment or be used after radiation therapy in cases where it was not successful.

One promising treatment, known as high-intensity focused ultrasound (HIFU), destroys cancer cells by heating them with highly focused ultrasonic beams. This treatment has been used more in Europe, but it is not commonly employed in the United States at this time. Studies are now under way to determine its safety and effectiveness.

Nutrition and lifestyle changes

A recent study found that in men with a rising PSA after surgery or radiation therapy, drinking pomegranate juice seemed to slow the time it took the PSA level to double. Larger studies are now under way to try to confirm these results.

Some encouraging early results have also been reported with flaxseed supplements. One small study in men with early prostate cancer found that daily flaxseed seemed to slow the rate at which prostate cancer cells multiplied. More research is needed to confirm this finding.

A recent report found that men who chose not to have treatment for their localized prostate cancer may be able to slow its growth with intensive lifestyle changes. The men ate a vegan diet (no meat, fish, eggs, or dairy products) and exercised frequently. They also took part in support groups and yoga. After one year the men saw, on average, a slight drop in their PSA level. It isn't known whether this effect will last since the report only followed the men for 1 year. The regimen may also be hard to follow for some men.

Hormone therapy

Even though LHRH analogs stop the testicles from making testosterone, the body can still make a small amount of androgens. A new drug, abiraterone, blocks an enzyme called CYP17, which is needed for the body to make many hormones, including androgens (such as testosterone). In an early study of men whose cancers were growing despite low testosterone levels (from LHRH analogs or orchiectomy), this drug lowered levels of androgens even more. It also shrank tumors and lowered PSA levels in these men, who had cancers that had stopped responding to hormone treatment. There were few side effects. Further studies are ongoing to see if this drug helps those with prostate cancer live longer.

Chemotherapy

Studies in recent years have shown that many chemotherapy drugs can affect prostate cancer. At least one drug, docetaxel (Taxotere), has been shown to help men live longer. Several new chemotherapy drugs and combinations of drugs are now being studied.

One drug that has been studied is satraplatin, which is taken in pill form. The drug was given to men with advanced, hormone-refractory prostate cancer whose cancer had already been treated with at least one chemotherapeutic drug. Although satraplatin did help keep the cancers from growing, it didn't appear to help the men live longer.

Calcitriol, a form of vitamin D, had shown promising results against hormone-refractory prostate cancer in an early study. The combination of calcitriol and docetaxel appeared to help men with advanced prostate cancer live longer than those who took docetaxel alone. Unfortunately, this finding was not confirmed by a larger clinical trial known as ASCENT2 (Androgen-independent prostate cancer Study of Calcitriol Enhancing Taxotere). In fact, in ASCENT2, the men who received calcitriol with docetaxel did not live as long as those who were treated with docetaxel and prednisone.

Prostate cancer vaccines

Several types of vaccines for boosting the body's immune response to prostate cancer cells are being tested in clinical trials. Unlike vaccines against infections like measles or mumps, these vaccines are designed to help treat, not prevent, prostate cancer. One possible advantage of these types of treatments is that they seem to have very limited side effects. One example of this type of vaccine is sipuleucel-T (Provenge).

Another prostate cancer vaccine (PROSTVAC-VF) uses a virus that has been genetically modified to contain prostate-specific antigen (PSA). The patient's immune system should respond to the virus and begin to recognize and destroy cancer cells containing PSA. This vaccine is still in early-stage clinical trials.

Several other prostate cancer vaccines are also in development.

Monoclonal antibodies

Monoclonal antibodies are man-made versions of immune system proteins designed to target specific molecules in prostate cancer cells or cells of the body that support cancer growth. Several different ones are being developed and tested.

When prostate cancer cells spread to the bones, the osteoclasts and osteoblasts (cells that the body uses to remodel bone) are turned on inappropriately. Denosumab is an antibody that blocks the osteoclasts from being turned on. Studies have shown that denosumab can help prevent and treat bone loss from treatment with hormone therapy in prostate cancer. The drug also appears to help men with bone metastases who are no longer helped by zoledronic acid (Zometa). Studies of denosumab are ongoing.

Angiogenesis inhibitors

Growth of prostate cancer tumors depends on growth of blood vessels (angiogenesis) to nourish the cancer cells. Looking at angiogenesis in prostate cancer specimens may help predict treatment outcomes. Cancers that stimulate many new vessels to grow are harder to treat and have a poorer outlook.

New drugs are being studied that may be useful in stopping prostate cancer growth by keeping new blood vessels from forming. Several anti-angiogenic drugs are already being tested in clinical trials. One of these is thalidomide, which has been approved by the U.S. Food and Drug Administration (FDA) to treat patients with multiple myeloma. It is being combined with chemotherapy in clinical trials to treat men with advanced prostate cancer. While promising, this drug can cause major side effects, including constipation, drowsiness, and nerve damage.

Another drug, bevacizumab (Avastin), is FDA-approved to treat patients with other cancers. It is now being tested in combination with hormone therapy and chemotherapy in men with advanced prostate cancer.

Treating bone pain

Doctors are now studying the use of radiofrequency ablation (RFA) to help control pain in men whose prostate cancer has spread to one or more areas in the bones. During RFA, the doctor uses computed tomography (CT) or ultrasound to guide a small metal probe into the area of the tumor. A high frequency current passed through the probe heats and destroys the tumor. RFA has been used for many years to treat tumors in other organs such as the liver, but its use in treating bone pain is still fairly new. Still, early results are promising.

Resources

Additional Resources

The American Cancer Society is happy to address any cancer-related topic. If you have questions, please call us at **800-227-2345**, 24 hours a day.

More Information from Your American Cancer Society

The following related materials may be ordered through our toll-free number: **800-227-2345**.

Spanish language versions of some of these documents are also available.

Caring for the Person with Cancer at Home: A Guide for Patients and Families

Guidelines for the Early Detection of Cancer

Managing Incontinence After Treatment for Prostate Cancer

Sexuality and Cancer: For the Man Who Has Cancer and His Partner

Understanding Chemotherapy: A Guide for Patients and Families

Understanding Radiation Therapy: A Guide for Patients and Families

National Organizations and Web Sites*

In addition to the American Cancer Society, the following other sources of patient information and support are available:

American Urological Association Foundation
Toll-free number: 866-746-4282 (866-RING-AUA)
Internet address: www.urologyhealth.org

National Association for Continence
Toll-free number: 800-252-3337 (800-BLADDER)
Internet address: www.nafc.org

National Cancer Institute
Toll-free number: 800-422-6237 (800-4-CANCER);
TYY: 800-332-8615
Internet address: www.cancer.gov

National Coalition for Cancer Survivorship
Toll-free number: 888-650-9127
877-622-7937 (877-NCCS-YES) for some
publications and Cancer Survivor Toolbox® orders
Internet address: www.canceradvocacy.org

**ZERO - The Project to End Prostate Cancer
(formerly National Prostate Cancer Coalition)**
Toll-free number: 888-245-9455
Internet address: www.zerocancer.org

Prostate Cancer Foundation (formerly "CaPCURE")
Toll-free number: 800-757-2873 (800-757-CURE)
or 310-570-4700
Internet address: www.pcf.org

US Too International, Inc.
Toll-free number: 800-808-7866 (800-80US TOO)
or 630-795-1002 (Chicago area)
Internet address: www.ustoo.com

---

*Inclusion on this list does not imply endorsement by the American Cancer Society.

No matter who you are, we can help. Contact us anytime, day or night, for information and support. Call us at **800-227-2345** or visit **cancer.org**.

References

Akaza H, Hinotsu S, Usami M, Arai Y, Kanetake H, Naito S, Hirao Y; Study Group for the Combined Androgen Blockade Therapy of Prostate Cancer. Combined androgen blockade with bicalutamide for advanced prostate cancer: long-term follow-up of a phase 3, double-blind, randomized study for survival. *Cancer.* 2009;115(15):3437–3445.

Algotar AM, Thompson PA, Ranger-Moore J, Stratton MS, Hsu CH, Ahmann FR, Nagle RB, Stratton SP. Effect of aspirin, other NSAIDs, and statins on PSA and PSA velocity. *Prostate.* 2010;70(8):883–888.

Altekruse SF, Kosary CL, Krapcho M, Neyman N, Aminou R, Waldron W, Ruhl J, Howlader N, Tatalovich Z, Cho H, Mariotto A, Eisner MP, Lewis DR, Cronin K, Chen HS, Feuer EJ, Stinchcomb DG, Edwards BK (eds). *SEER Cancer Statistics Review, 1975–2007,* National Cancer Institute. Bethesda, MD, http://seer.cancer.gov/csr/1975_2007/, based on November 2009 SEER data submission, posted to the SEER Web site, 2010.

American Cancer Society. *Cancer Facts and Figures 2010.* Atlanta, GA: American Cancer Society; 2010.

American Joint Committee on Cancer. Prostate. In: *AJCC Cancer Staging Manual.* 7th ed. New York: Springer; 2010:457–464.

Andriole GL, Bostwick DG, Brawley OW, Gomella LG, Marberger M, Montorsi F, Pettaway CA, Tammela TL, Teloken C, Tindall DJ, Somerville MC, Wilson TH, Fowler IL, Rittmaster RS; REDUCE Study Group. Effect of dutasteride on the risk of prostate cancer. *N Engl J Med.* 2010;362(13):1192–1202.

Andriole GL, Crawford ED, Grubb RL 3rd, Buys SS, Chia D, Church TR, Fouad MN, Gelmann EP, Kvale PA, Reding DJ, Weissfeld JL, Yokuchi LA, O'Brien B, Clapp JD, Rathmell JM, Riley TL, Hayes RB, Kramer BS, Izmirlian G, Miller AB, Pinsky PF, Prorok PC, Gohagan JK, Berg CD; PLCO Project Team. Mortality results from a randomized prostate-cancer screening trial. *N Engl J Med.* 2009;360(13):1310–1319. Epub 2009 Mar 18.

Attard G, Reid AHM, Yap TA, Raynaud F, Dowsett M, Settatree S, Barrett M, Parker C, Martins V, Folkerd E, Clark J, Cooper CS, Kaye SB, Dearnaley D, Lee G, de Bono JS. Phase I clinical trial of a selective inhibitor of CYP17, abiraterone acetate, confirms that castration-resistant prostate cancer commonly remains hormone driven. *J Clin Oncol.* 2008;26(28):4563–4571. Epub 2008 Jul 21.

Barnas JL, Pierpaoli S, Ladd P, Valenzuela R, Aviv N, Parker M, Waters WB, Flanigan FC, Mulhall JP. The prevalence and nature of orgasmic dysfunction after radical prostatectomy. *BJU Int.* 2004;94(4):603–605.

Beer TM, Ryan CW, Venner PM, Petrylak DP, Chatta GS, Ruether JD, Redfern CH, Fehrenbacher L, Saleh MN, Waterhouse DM, Carducci MA, Vicario D, Dreicer R, Higano CS, Ahmann FR, Chi KN, Henner WD, Arroyo A, Clow FW. A Report from the ASCENT Investigators. Double-blinded randomized study of high-dose calcitriol plus docetaxel compared with placebo plus docetaxel in androgen-independent prostate cancer: a report from the ASCENT Investigators. *J Clin Oncol.* 2007;25(6):669–674.

Bostwick DG, Crawford ED, Higano CS, Roach M III, eds. *American Cancer Society's Complete Guide to Prostate Cancer.* Atlanta, GA: American Cancer Society; 2005.

Danila DC, Morris MJ, de Bono JS, Ryan CJ, Denmeade SR, Smith MR, Taplin ME, Bubley GJ, Kheoh T,

Hagg C, Molina A, Anand A, Koscuiszka M, Larson SM, Schwartz LH, Fleisher M, Scher HI. Phase II multicenter study of abiraterone acetate plus prednisone therapy in patients with docetaxel-treated castration-resistant prostate cancer. *J Clin Oncol.* 2010;28(9):1496–1501.

De Bono JS, Oudard S, Ozguroglu M, Hansen S, Machiels H, Shen L, Matthews P, Sartor AO, for the TROPIC Investigators. Cabazitaxel or mitoxantrone with prednisone in patients with metastatic castration-resistant prostate cancer (mCRPC) previously treated with docetaxel: Final results of a multinational phase III trial (TROPIC). *J Clin Oncol* 2010;(Suppl:Abstract 4508). ASCO Meeting Abstracts May 20, 2010:4508.

Epstein JI. An update of the Gleason grading system. *J Urol.* 2010;183(2):433–440. Epub 2009 Dec 14.

Fizazi K, Bosserman L, Gao G, Skacel T, Markus R. Denosumab treatment of prostate cancer with bone metastases and increased urine N-telopeptide levels after therapy with intravenous bisphosphonates: results of a randomized phase II trial. *J Urol.* 2009;182(2):509–515. Epub 2009 Jun 13.

Giovanucci E, Platz EA. Epidemiology of prostate cancer. In: Vogelzang NJ, Scardino PT, Shipley WU, Debruyne FMJ, Linehan WM, eds. *Comprehensive Textbook of Genitourinary Oncology.* 3rd ed. Philadelphia, PA: Lippincott Williams & Wilkins; 2006:9–21.

Hamilton A, Ries LAG. Cancer of the prostate. In: Ries LAG, Young JL Jr, Keel GE, Eisner MP, Lin YD, Horner MJ-D, eds. *SEER Survival Monograph: Cancer Survival Among Adults: U.S. SEER Program, 1988-2001, Patient and Tumor Characteristics.* National Cancer Institute, SEER Program, NIH Pub. No. 07-6215, Bethesda, MD, 2007.

Higano CS, Schellhammer PF, Small EJ, Burch PA, Nemunaitis J, Yuh L, Provost N, Frohlich MW.

Integrated data from 2 randomized, double-blind, placebo-controlled, phase 3 trials of active cellular immunotherapy with sipuleucel-T in advanced prostate cancer. *Cancer.* 2009;115(16):3670–3679.

Hugosson J, Carlsson S, Aus G, Bergdahl S, Khatami A, Lodding P, Pihl CG, Stranne J, Holmberg E, Lilja H. Mortality results from the Göteborg randomised population-based prostate-cancer screening trial. *Lancet Oncol.* 2010;11(8):725–732. Epub 2010 Jul 2 [ahead of print].

Huncharek M, Haddock KS, Reid R, Kupelnick B. Smoking as a risk factor for prostate cancer: a meta-analysis of 24 prospective cohort studies. *Am J Public Health.* 2010;100(4):693–701. Epub 2009 Jul 16.

Kyrgidis A, Vahtsevanos K, Koloutsos G, Andreadis C, Boukovinas I, Teleioudis Z, Patrikidou A, Triaridis S. Bisphosphonate-related osteonecrosis of the jaws: A case-control study of risk factors in breast cancer patients. *J Clin Oncol.* 2008;26(28):4634–4638. Epub 2008 Jun 23.

Lin DW. Beyond PSA: utility of novel tumor markers in the setting of elevated PSA. *Urol Oncol.* 2009;27(3):315–321.

Lippman SM, Klein EA, Goodman PJ, Lucia MS, Thompson IM, Ford LG, Parnes HL, Minasian LM, Gaziano JM, Hartline JA, Parsons JK, Bearden JD 3rd, Crawford ED, Goodman GE, Claudio J, Winquist E, Cook ED, Karp DD, Walther P, Lieber MM, Kristal AR, Darke AK, Arnold KB, Ganz PA, Santella RM, Albanes D, Taylor PR, Probstfield JL, Jagpal TJ, Crowley JJ, Meyskens FL Jr, Baker LH, Coltman CA Jr. Effect of selenium and vitamin E on risk of prostate cancer and other cancers: the Selenium and Vitamin E Cancer Prevention Trial (SELECT). *JAMA.* 2009;301(1):39–51. Epub 2008 Dec 9.

Lu-Yao GL, Albertsen PC, Moore DF, Shih W, Lin Y, DiPaola RS, Yao S-L. Survival following primary androgen deprivation therapy among men with localized prostate cancer. *JAMA*. 2008;300(2): 173–181.

Lucia MS, Epstein JI, Goodman PJ, Darke AK, Reuter VE, Civantos F, Tangen CM, Parnes HL, Lippman SM, La Rosa FG, Kattan MW, Crawford ED, Ford LG, Coltman CA Jr, Thompson IM. Finasteride and high-grade prostate cancer in the Prostate Cancer Prevention Trial. *J Natl Cancer Inst*. 2007;99(18):1375–1383. Epub 2007 Sep 11.

Nanda A, Chen MH, Moran BJ, Braccioforte MH, Dosoretz D, Salenius S, Katin M, Ross R, D'Amico AV. Total androgen blockade versus a luteinizing hormone-releasing hormone agonist alone in men with high-risk prostate cancer treated with radiotherapy. *Int J Radiat Oncol Biol Phys*. 2010;76(5):1439–1444. Epub 2009 Jun 18.

National Cancer Institute. Physician Data Query (PDQ). *Prostate Cancer: Treatment*. 2010. National Cancer Institute Web site. www.cancer.gov/cancertopics/pdq/treatment/prostate/healthprofessional. Accessed on June 9, 2010.

National Comprehensive Cancer Network (NCCN). *Practice Guidelines in Oncology: Prostate Cancer. Version 2.2010*. National Comprehensive Cancer Network Web site. www.nccn.org. Accessed on June 8, 2010.

Nelson CJ, Lee JS, Gamboa MC, Roth AJ. Cognitive effects of hormone therapy in men with prostate cancer: a review. *Cancer*. 2008;113(5):1097–1106.

Nelson WG, Carter HB, DeWeese TL, et al. Prostate cancer. In: Abeloff MD, Armitage JO, Lichter AS, Niederhuber JE. Kastan MB, McKenna WG, eds. *Clinical Oncology*. 4th ed. Philadelphia, PA: Elsevier; 2008:1653–1699.

Ornish D, Weidner G, Fair WR, Marlin R, Pettengill EB, Raisin CJ, Dunn-Emke S, Crutchfield L, Jacobs FN, Barnard RJ, Aronson WJ, McCormac P, McKnight DJ, Fein JD, Dnistrian AM, Weinstein J, Ngo TH, Mendell NR, Carroll PR. Intensive lifestyle changes may affect the progression of prostate cancer. *J Urol.* 2005;174(3):1065–1069; discussion 1069–1070.

Potosky AL, Davis WW, Hoffman RM, Stanford JL, Stephenson RA, Penson DF, Harlan LC. Five-year outcomes after prostatectomy or radiotherapy for prostate cancer: The Prostate Cancer Outcomes Study. *J Natl Cancer Inst.* 2004;96(18):1358–1367.

Pound CR, Partin AW, Eisenberger MA, Chan DW, Pearson JD, Walsh PC. Natural history of progression after PSA elevation following radical prostatectomy. *JAMA.* 1999;281(17):1591–1597.

Price MM, Hamilton RJ, Robertson CN, Butts MC, Freedland SJ. Body mass index, prostate-specific antigen, and digital rectal examination findings among participants in a prostate cancer screening clinic. *Urology.* 2008;71(5):787–791. Epub 2008 Feb 11.

Quinlan DM, Epstein JI, Carter BS, Walsh PC. Sexual function following radical prostatectomy: influence of preservation of neurovascular bundles. *J Urol.* 1991;145(5):998–1002.

Ryan CJ, Smith MR, Fong L, Rosenberg JE, Kantoff P, Raynaud F, Martins V, Lee G, Kheoh T, Kim J, Molina A, Small EJ. Phase I clinical trial of the CYP17 inhibitor abiraterone acetate demonstrating clinical activity in patients with castration-resistant prostate cancer who received prior ketoconazole therapy. *J Clin Oncol.* 2010;28(9):1481–1488. Epub 2010 Feb 16.

Savoie M, Kim SS, Soloway MS. A prospective study measuring penile length in men treated with radical prostatectomy for prostate cancer. *J Urol.* 2003;169(4):1462–1464.

Scher HI, Chi KN, De Wit R, Berry WR, Albers P, Henick B, Venner P, Heidenreich A, Chu L, Heller G. Docetaxel (D) plus high dose calcitriol versus D plus prednisone (P) for patients (Pts) with progressive castration-resistant prostate cancer (CRPC): Results from the phase III ASCENT2 trial. *J Clin Oncol.* 2010(Suppl:Abstract 4509). ASCO Annual Meeting Abstracts May 20, 2010:4509.

Schröder FH, Hugosson J, Roobol MJ, Tammela TLJ, Ciatto S, Nelen V, Kwiatkowski M, Lujan M, Lilja H, Zappa M, Denis LJ, Recker F, Berenguer A, Määttänen L, Bangma CH, Aus G, Villers A, Rebillard X, van der Kwast T, Blijenberg BG, Moss SM, de Koning HJ, Auvinen A; ERSPC Investigators. Screening and prostate-cancer mortality in a randomized European study. *N Engl J Med.* 2009;360(13):1320–1328. Epub 2009 Mar 18.

Shinohara K, Master VA, Chi T, Carroll PR. Prostate needle biopsy techniques and interpretation. In: Vogelzang NJ, Scardino PT, Shipley WU, Debruyne FMJ, Linehan WM, eds. *Comprehensive Textbook of Genitourinary Oncology.* 3rd ed. Philadelphia, PA: Lippincott Williams & Wilkins; 2006:111–119.

Smith MR, Egerdie B, Hernández Toriz N, Feldman R, Tammela TL, Saad F, Heracek J, Szwedowski M, Ke C, Kupic A, Leder BZ, Goessl C; Denosumab HALT Prostate Cancer Study Group. Denosumab in men receiving androgen-deprivation therapy for prostate cancer. *N Engl J Med.* 2009;361(8):745–755.

Sternberg CN, Petrylak DP, Sartor O, Witjes JA, Demkow T, Ferrero JM, Eymard JC, Falcon S, Calabrò F, James N, Bodrogi I, Harper P, Wirth M, Berry W, Petrone ME, McKearn TJ, Noursalehi M, George M, Rozencweig M. Multinational, double-blind, phase III study of prednisone and either satraplatin or placebo in patients with castrate-refractory prostate cancer progressing after prior chemotherapy: the SPARC trial. *J Clin Oncol.* 2009;27(32):5431–5438. Epub 2009 Oct 5.

Sun M, Lughezzani G, Alasker A, Isbarn H, Jeldres C, Shariat SF, Budäus L, Lattouf JB, Valiquette L, Graefen M, Montorsi F, Perrotte P, Karakiewicz PI. Comparative study of inguinal hernia repair after radical prostatectomy, prostate biopsy, transurethral resection of the prostate or pelvic lymph node dissection. *J Urol.* 2010;183(3):970–975. Epub 2010 Jan 18.

Wolf AMD, Wender RC, Etzioni RB, Thompson IM, D'Amico AV, Volk RJ, Brooks DD, Dash C, Guessous I, Andrews K, Desantis C, Smith RA. American Cancer Society Guideline for the Early Detection of Prostate Cancer: Update 2010. *CA Cancer J Clin.* 2010;60(2):70-98. Epub 2010 Mar 3.

Zelefsky MJ, Eastham JA, Sartor OA, Kantoff P. Cancer of the prostate. In: DeVita VT Jr, Lawrence TS, Rosenberg SA, eds. *DeVita, Hellman, and Rosenberg's Cancer: Principles and Practice of Oncology.* 8th ed. Philadelphia, PA: Lippincott Williams & Wilkins; 2008:1392–1452.

Glossary

active surveillance: *see* watchful waiting.

adenocarcinoma (add-uh-no-kahr-si-NO-muh): cancer that starts in the glandular tissue, such as in the prostate. *See also* gland.

alternative therapy (alternative medicine): use of an unproven therapy instead of standard (proven) therapy. Some alternative therapies may have dangerous or even life-threatening side effects. For others, the main danger is that a patient may lose the opportunity to benefit from standard therapy. The Society recommends that patients considering use of any alternative or complementary therapy discuss this with their health care team. *See also* complementary therapy.

androgen (AN-droh-jen): any male sex hormone. The major androgen is testosterone.

androgen deprivation therapy (AN-droh-jen DEH-prih-VAY-shun THAYR-uh-pee) (ADT): Also called androgen suppression therapy. *See* hormone therapy.

androgen-independent: term for prostate cancer cells that no longer respond to hormone therapy. Also called hormone-refractory. *Compare with* androgen-dependent.

anesthesia (an-es-THEE-zhuh): the loss of feeling or sensation as a result of drugs or gases. **General anesthesia** causes loss of consciousness (makes you go into a deep sleep). **Local** or **regional anesthesia** numbs only a certain area of the body. **Epidural anesthesia** uses an injection of anesthetic drugs into the space around the spinal cord in order to numb the lower part of the body while allowing the patient to remain awake.

anesthetic (an-es-THEH-tik): a topical or intravenous substance that causes loss of feeling or awareness in a part of the body. General anesthetics are used to put patients to sleep for procedures. *See also* anesthesia.

antiandrogen (AN-tee-AN-droh-jen): a drug used to block the production or interfere with the action of male sex hormones. Antiandrogens are usually used in combination with orchiectomy or LHRH analogs. Several drugs of this type are currently available—flutamide (Eulexin), bicalutamide (Casodex), and nilutamide (Nilandron).

artificial sphincter: an inflatable cuff implanted around the upper urethra to squeeze the urethra shut and provide urinary control.

atypia (ay-TIH-pee-uh): the appearance of cancerous or precancerous cells. *See also* hyperplasia.

atypical small acinar proliferation (ASAP): prostate cells that look like they might be cancerous, but there are too few cells in the biopsy sample to be sure. With ASAP, there's about a 40% to 50% chance of prostate cancer, so many doctors advise a repeat biopsy within a few months. Also called atypia.

benign: not cancer; not malignant.

benign prostatic hyperplasia (beh-NINE prah-STA-tik HY-per-PLAY-zhuh) (BPH): noncancerous enlargement of the prostate that may cause problems with urination such as trouble starting and stopping the flow. Also referred to as BPH.

biopsy (BUY-op-see): the removal of a sample of tissue to see whether cancer cells are present. There are several kinds of biopsies. In a fine needle aspiration biopsy (sometimes used to check pelvic lymph nodes), a very thin needle is used to draw out fluid and cells. In a core biopsy, a larger needle is used to remove a thin cylinder of tissue. In a sextant biopsy, six core biopsy samples are taken, one each from the top, middle, and bottom of each side of the prostate.

bisphosphonates (bis-FOS-foh-nayts): drugs that are sometimes given to cancer patients whose disease has spread to the bones. When injected into a vein or taken by mouth, bisphosphonates can slow the breakdown of bone, lower the rate of bone fractures, and treat bone pain. Bisphosphonates are most commonly used in breast cancer and multiple myeloma (a type of bone cancer), but are now approved for use in men with prostate cancer that has spread to the bones.

bladder: a hollow organ with flexible, muscular walls that stores urine.

bone scan: an imaging method that gives important information about the bones, including the location of cancer that may have spread to the bones. It can be done as an outpatient procedure and is painless, except for the needle stick when a low-dose radioactive substance is injected into a vein. Special pictures are taken to see where the radioactivity collects, pointing to an abnormality.

BPH: *see* benign prostatic hyperplasia.

brachytherapy (brake-ee-THAYR-uh-pee): internal radiation treatment given by placing radioactive material directly into the tumor or close to it. Also called interstitial radiation therapy or seed implantation. *Compare with* external beam radiation therapy. *See also* interstitial radiation therapy.

BRCA1: a gene on chromosome 17 that normally helps to suppress cell growth. A person who inherits certain mutations (changes) in a BRCA1 gene has a higher risk of getting breast, ovarian, prostate, and other types of cancer.

BRCA2: a gene on chromosome 13 that normally helps to suppress cell growth. A person who inherits certain mutations (changes) in a BRCA2 gene has a higher risk of getting breast, ovarian, prostate, and other types of cancer.

cancer: cancer is not just one disease but a group of diseases. All forms of cancer cause cells in the body to change and grow out of control. Most types of cancer cells form a lump or mass called a tumor. The tumor can invade and destroy healthy tissue. Cells from the tumor can break away and travel to other parts of the body. There they can continue to grow. This spreading process is called metastasis. When cancer spreads, it is still named after the part of the body where it started. For example, if breast cancer spreads to the lungs, it is still called breast cancer, not lung cancer.

Some cancers, such as blood cancers, do not form a tumor. Not all tumors are cancer. A tumor that is not cancer is called **benign**. Benign tumors do not grow and spread the way cancer does. Benign tumors are usually not a threat to life. Another word for cancerous is **malignant**.

cancer care team: the group of health care professionals who work together to find, treat, and care for people with cancer. The cancer care team may include the following and others: primary care physicians, pathologists, oncology specialists (medical oncologist, radiation oncologist), surgeons (including surgical specialists such as urologists, gynecologists, neurosurgeons, etc.), nurses, oncology nurse specialists, and oncology social workers. Whether the team is linked formally or informally, there is usually one person who takes the job of coordinating the team.

cancer cell: a cell that divides and reproduces abnormally and has the potential to spread throughout the body, crowding out normal cells and tissue. *See also* metastasis.

castration: surgery to remove the testicles; Also called orchiectomy. *Compare with* chemical castration.

catheter (CATH-uh-tur): a thin, flexible tube through which fluids enter or leave the body; for example, a tube inserted through the tip of the penis into the bladder to drain urine (known as a Foley catheter).

cell: the basic unit of which all living things are made. Cells replace themselves by splitting and forming new cells (mitosis). The processes that control the formation of new cells and the death of old cells are disrupted in cancer.

chemical castration: the use of hormone therapy medications to achieve very low levels of testosterone without surgical removal of the testicles. *Compare with* castration, orchiectomy.

chemotherapy (key-mo-THAYR-uh-pee): treatment with drugs to destroy cancer cells. Chemotherapy is often used, either alone or with surgery or radiation, to treat cancer that has spread or come back (recurred), or when there is a strong chance that it could recur.

clinical stage: an estimate of the extent of cancer based on physical exam, biopsy results, and imaging tests. *See also* pathologic stage, staging.

clinical trials: research studies to test new drugs or other treatments to compare current, standard treatments with others that may be better. Before a new treatment is used on people, it is studied in the laboratory. If laboratory studies suggest the treatment will work, the next step is to test its value for patients. These human studies are called clinical trials.

combination hormone therapy: *see* combined androgen blockade.

combined androgen blockade (CAB): complete blockage of androgen production that may include castration (orchiectomy) or LHRH analogs, plus the use of antiandrogens. Also called combination hormone therapy, total hormonal ablation, total androgen blockade, or total androgen ablation.

complementary therapy (complementary medicine): treatment used in addition to standard therapy. Some complementary therapies may help relieve certain symptoms of cancer, relieve side effects of standard cancer therapy, or improve a patient's sense of well-being. The American Cancer Society recommends that patients considering the use of any alternative or complementary therapies discuss these therapies with their cancer care team, since many of these treatments are unproven and some can be harmful. *Compare with* alternative therapy.

complexed PSA: the portion of PSA that is not "free," that is, the part that is not bound to proteins. Researchers are studying whether measuring this, rather than total PSA, may give a more accurate picture of whether prostate cancer is present. *See also* prostate-specific antigen, free-PSA ratio.

computed tomography (to-MAHG-ruh-fee): an imaging test in which many x-rays are taken of a part of the body from different angles. These images are combined by a computer to produce cross-sectional pictures of internal organs. Except for the injection of a contrast dye (needed in some but not all cases), this procedure is painless and can be done in an outpatient clinic. It is often referred to as "CT" or "CAT" scanning.

contrast solution: any material used in imaging tests, such as x-rays and MRI and CT scans, to help outline the body parts being examined. These solutions may be injected or ingested (drunk). Also called contrast dye, contrast material. *See also* imaging tests.

cryoablation (kry-oh-ab-LAY-shun): use of extreme cold to freeze and destroy cancer cells.

cryosurgery: *see* cryoablation.

CT scan or **CAT scan:** *see* computed tomography.

curative treatment: treatment aimed at producing a cure. *Compare with* palliative treatment.

diagnosis: identifying a disease by its signs or symptoms and by using imaging procedures and laboratory findings. For some types of cancer, the earlier a diagnosis is made, the better the chance for long-term survival.

digital rectal examination (DRE): an examination during which the doctor inserts a lubricated, gloved finger into the rectum to feel for anything abnormal. Some tumors of the rectum and prostate gland can be felt during this examination.

dihydrotestosterone (die-hi-dro-tes-TOSS-ter-own) (DHT): a powerful form of male hormone produced by the action of 5-alpha reductase (a prostate enzyme) on testosterone. *See also* 5-alpha reductase.

distant stage: *see* staging.

DNA: deoxyribonucleic acid. DNA is the genetic "blueprint" found in the nucleus of each cell. It holds genetic information on cell growth, division, and function.

DRE: *see* digital rectal examination.

early detection: use of routine screening tests to try and detect cancer before it causes symptoms. The PSA is often used in this way. *See* screening and prostate-specific antigen.

erectile dysfunction: not being able to have or keep an erection of the penis. Also called impotence.

estrogen (ES-truh-jin): a female sex hormone produced mainly by the ovaries, and in smaller amounts by the adrenal glands. It is sometimes given to men with advanced prostate cancer to counteract the action of testosterone.

expectant management: *see* watchful waiting.

external beam radiation therapy: radiation that is focused on the area affected by cancer from a source outside the body. It is much like getting a diagnostic x-ray, but for a longer time and at a higher dose. *Compare with* brachytherapy.

false negative: test result implying a condition does not exist when, in fact, it does. *Compare with* false positive.

false positive: test result implying a condition exists when, in fact, it does not. *Compare with* false negative.

fatigue (fuh-TEEG): a common symptom during cancer treatment, a bone-weary exhaustion that doesn't get better with rest. For some, this condition can last for some time after treatment.

FDA: *see* U.S. Food and Drug Administration.

fine needle aspiration (FNA) biopsy: a procedure in which a thin needle is used to draw up (aspirate) samples for examination under a microscope. *See also* biopsy.

5-alpha reductase (5-AL-fuh ree-DUK-tays): an enzyme that converts testosterone to a more active hormone called dihydrotestosterone (DHT). Drugs such a finasteride (Proscar or Propecia) that prevent this conversion are called 5-alpha reductase inhibitors and may help reduce the risk of prostate cancer. *See also* dihydrotestosterone.

five (5)-year relative survival rate: the percentage of people with a certain cancer who have not died of it within 5 years. This number is different from the 5-year survival rate in that it does not include people who have died of unrelated causes. Relative survival rates are important for prostate cancer because many men with it are older and may die of other health problems. *Compare with* five-year survival rate.

five (5)-year survival rate: the percentage of people with a given cancer who are expected to survive 5 years or longer with the disease. Five-year survival rates have some drawbacks. Although the rates are based on the most recent information available, they may include data from patients treated several years earlier. Advances in cancer treatment often occur quickly. Five-year survival rates, while statistically valid, may not reflect these advances. They should not be seen as a predictor in an individual case. *Compare with* five (5)-year relative survival rate.

frozen section: a very thin slice of tissue that has been quick-frozen and then examined under a microscope. This method is sometimes used during an operation because it allows for a quick diagnosis. The surgeon can then determine whether or not to continue with the procedure. The diagnosis is confirmed in a few days by a more detailed study called a **permanent section**.

gene: a segment of DNA that contains information on hereditary characteristics such as hair color, eye color, and height, as well as susceptibility to certain diseases. *See also* DNA.

gland: a cell or group of cells that produce and release substances used nearby or in another part of the body. The prostate is an example of a gland.

Gleason grade: the most often used prostate cancer grading system is called the **Gleason system**. A pathologist assigns a Gleason grade ranging from 1 through 5 based on how much the cancer cells under the microscope look like normal prostate cells. Those that look a lot like normal cells are graded as 1, while those that look the least like normal cells are graded as 5. *See also* Gleason score, grade.

Gleason score: the combined total of the two Gleason grades used in classifying each prostate cancer, based on how the cells appear under the microscope. Because prostate cancers often have areas with different grades, a grade is assigned to the two areas that make up most of the cancer. These two grades are added together to give a Gleason score between 2 and 10. The higher the Gleason score, the faster the cancer is likely to grow and the more likely it is to spread beyond the prostate. Also called the Gleason sum.

Gleason system: the most often used prostate cancer grading system. A pathologist assigns a Gleason grade ranging from 1 through 5 based on how much the cancer cells under the microscope look like normal prostate cells. Those that look a lot like normal cells are graded as 1, while those that look the least like normal cells are graded as 5. Prostate cancer often has areas with different grades and more than one grade may apply. *See also* Gleason score, Gleason grade, grade.

grade: the grade of a cancer reflects how abnormal it looks under the microscope. There are several grading systems for different types of cancers, such as the Gleason system for prostate cancer. Each grading system divides cancer into those with the greatest abnormality, the least abnormality, and those in between.

Grading is done by a pathologist who examines the tissue from the biopsy. It is important because cancers with more abnormal-appearing cells tend to grow and spread more quickly and have a worse prognosis (outlook). *See also* differentiation, Gleason grade, Gleason score, Gleason system, grade, prognosis.

hematuria (HEE-muh-TOOR-ee-uh): the presence of blood in the urine.

high dose rate (HDR) brachytherapy (brake-ee-THAYR-uh-pee): a form of treatment involving insertion of small plastic catheters into the prostate gland, guided by transrectal ultrasound (TRUS). A radioactive source (iridium-192) is then placed in the catheters and is removed a short time later. It is usually given once a week for 2 or 3 weeks and is often used in combination with external beam radiation therapy. Unlike standard brachytherapy (which uses lower doses of radiation over a longer period of time), the radioactive seeds are not left in the body.

hormone: a chemical substance released into the body by the endocrine glands such as the thyroid, adrenal, or ovaries. Hormones travel through the bloodstream and set in motion various body functions. Testosterone and estrogen are examples of male and female hormones.

hormone therapy: treatment with hormones using drugs that interfere with hormone production or hormone action, or the surgical removal of hormone-producing glands. Hormone therapy may kill cancer cells or slow their growth. It is a common form of treatment for advanced prostate cancer. *See also* hormone.

hospice: a special kind of care for people in the final phase of illness, their families, and caregivers. The care may take place in the patient's home or in a home-like facility.

HPC1 (Hereditary Prostate Cancer Gene 1): a gene linked to some cases of prostate cancer. Inherited DNA changes in HPC1 may make prostate cancer more likely to develop in some men. These changes appear to be responsible for about 10% of prostate cancers. Research on this gene is still preliminary, and a genetic test is not yet available.

imaging tests: methods used to produce pictures of internal body structures. Some imaging methods used to help diagnose or stage cancer are x-rays, CT scans, magnetic resonance imaging (MRI), and ultrasound.

impotence: not being able to have or maintain an erection of the penis. Also called erectile dysfunction.

incision (in-SIH-zhun): a cut made during surgery.

incontinence (in-KAHN-tih-nens): partial or complete loss of urinary control. **Urge incontinence** refers to a sudden and uncontrollable urge to pass urine. This problem occurs when the bladder becomes too sensitive to stretching by urine accumulation. **Overflow incontinence** refers to the need to get up often during the night to urinate, to take a long time to urinate, and to have a dribbling stream with little force. Overflow incontinence is usually due to blockage or narrowing of the bladder outlet, either from cancer or scar tissue. **Stress incontinence** refers to passing a small amount of urine when coughing, laughing, sneezing, or exercising.

insulin-like growth factor-1 (IGF-1): a hormone-like substance believed to affect growth hormone activity. Researchers have recently noted that men with high blood levels of IGF-1 may be more likely to have prostate cancer develop.

intensity modulated radiation therapy (IMRT): an advanced method of conformal radiation therapy in which the beams are aimed from several directions and the intensity (strength) of the beams is controlled by computers. This technique allows more radiation to reach the treatment area while reducing the damage to healthy tissues. *See also* three-dimensional conformal radiation therapy.

intermittent hormone therapy: a type of prostate cancer treatment in which hormonal drugs are stopped after a man's blood prostate-specific antigen (PSA) level drops to a very low level and remains stable for a while. If the PSA level begins to rise, the drugs are started again.

internal radiation therapy: treatment involving implantation of a radioactive substance into the body. *See also* brachytherapy.

interstitial radiation (in-ter-STIH-shul RAY-dee-AY-shun) therapy: a type of treatment in which a radioactive implant is placed directly into the tissue.

intravenous (in-tra-VEEN-us) (IV) line: a method of supplying fluids and medications by using a needle or a thin tube inserted in a vein.

isoflavones: sometimes called phytoestrogens, or plant estrogens, these compounds act like weak forms of estrogen but are not produced by the body. They are found in soy and other foods. *See also* estrogen.

Kegel exercises: exercises to strengthen bladder muscles. These exercises may help men and women with certain forms of incontinence.

laparoscope (LA-puh-ruh-SKOPE): a long, slender tube inserted into the abdomen through a very small incision. The laparoscope allows the surgeon to view organs and lymph nodes within the body. The lymph nodes, or even the prostate gland itself, can be removed by using special surgical instruments operated through the laparoscope.

laparoscopic radical prostatectomy (LRP): a surgical procedure in which the prostate is removed by using a laparoscope. This procedure is still widely considered to be experimental.

LHRH analogs: man-made hormones, chemically similar to luteinizing hormone-releasing hormone (LHRH). They block the production of the male hormone testosterone and are sometimes used as a treatment for prostate cancer. LHRH analogs approved for use in the United States include leuprolide, goserelin, and triptorelin. Also called LHRH agonists.

local stage (or localized cancer): *see* staging.

luteinizing (LOO-tih-NY-zing) hormone-releasing hormone (LHRH): a hormone produced by the hypothalamus, a tiny gland in the brain, that affects levels of luteinizing hormone (LH) in the body and therefore affects testosterone levels.

lycopenes (LIE-kuh-peens): vitamin-like antioxidants that help prevent damage to DNA and may help lower prostate cancer risk. These substances are found in tomatoes, pink grapefruit, and watermelon.

lymphadenectomy (lim-fad-uh-NECK-tuh-me): surgical removal of one or more lymph nodes. After removal, the lymph nodes are examined under a microscope to see if cancer is present. Also called lymph node dissection. *See also* lymph nodes, lymphedema.

lymphedema (limf-uh-DEE-muh): swelling due to a collection of excess fluid. This condition may occur soon after the lymph nodes and vessels are removed or are injured by radiation, or many years after treatment. It may also occur when a tumor disrupts normal fluid drainage. Lymphedema can persist and interfere with activities of daily living. *See also* lymph nodes, lymphadenectomy.

lymph nodes: small bean-shaped collections of immune system tissue such as lymphocytes, found along lymphatic vessels. They remove cell waste, germs, and other harmful substances from lymph. They help fight infections and also have a role in fighting cancer, although cancers sometimes spread through lymph nodes. Also called lymph glands. *See also* lymphadenectomy.

magnetic resonance imaging (MRI): a method of taking pictures of the inside of the body. Instead of using x-rays, MRI uses a powerful magnet to send radio waves through the body. The images appear on a computer screen, as well as on film. Like x-rays, the procedure is physically painless, but some people may feel confined inside the MRI machine.

malignant: cancerous.

malignant tumor: a mass of cancer cells that may invade surrounding tissues or spread (metastasize) to distant sites in the body. *See also* tumor, metastasis.

metastasis (meh-TAS-teh-sis): cancer cells that have spread to one or more sites elsewhere in the body, often by way of the lymphatic system or bloodstream. Regional metastasis is cancer that has spread to the lymph nodes, tissues, or organs close to the primary site. Distant metastasis is cancer that has spread to organs or tissues that are farther away (such as when colon cancer spreads to the lungs or liver). The plural of this word is metastases. *See also* metastasize, metastatic.

metastatic (met-uh-STAT-ick) cancer: a way to describe cancer that has spread from the primary site (where it started) to other structures or organs, nearby or far away (distant). *See also* metastasis.

metastasize (meh-TAS-tuh-size): the spread of cancer cells to one or more sites elsewhere in the body, often by way of the lymphatic system or bloodstream. *See also* metastasis, metastatic.

monoclonal (ma-nuh-KLO-nuhl) antibody: a man-made antibody that is designed to lock onto certain antigens. Antigens are substances that can be recognized by the immune system. Monoclonal antibodies (MAbs) have several uses in cancer and its treatment. Monoclonal antibodies that have been attached to chemotherapy drugs or radioactive substances are able to seek out antigens unique to cancer cells and deliver these treatments directly to the cancer, thus killing the cancer cell and not harming healthy tissue. "Naked" monoclonal antibodies can attach to cancer cells so that the cancer cells can be found and attacked by the body. Research is still going on to learn more ways they can be used to treat cancer. Monoclonal antibodies are also often used to help detect and classify cancer cells under a microscope. Other studies are being done to see if radioactive atoms attached to monoclonal antibodies can be used in imaging tests to detect and locate small groups of cancer cells.

MRI: *see* magnetic resonance imaging.

mutation (myoo-TAY-shun): a change in the DNA of a cell. Most mutations do not produce cancer, and a few may even be helpful. However, all types of cancer are thought to be due to mutations that damage a cell's DNA. Some cancer-related mutations can be inherited, which means that the person is born with the mutated DNA in all the body's cells. But most mutations happen after the person is born, and are called somatic mutations. This type of mutation happens in one cell at a time, and only affects cells that arise from the single mutated cell. *See also* DNA.

oncogenes (ON-koh-jeens): genes that promote cell growth and multiplication. These genes are normally present in all cells. But oncogenes may undergo changes that activate them, causing cells to grow too quickly and form tumors.

orchiectomy (or-kee-EK-toh-mee): surgery to remove the testicles. Also called castration. *Compare with* chemical castration.

palliative (PAL-ee-uh-tiv) treatment: treatment that relieves symptoms, such as pain or blockage of urine flow, but is not expected to cure the disease. Its main purpose is to improve the patient's quality of life. Sometimes chemotherapy and radiation are used as palliative treatments. *Compare with* curative treatment.

pathologic stage: an estimate of the extent of cancer by direct study of the tissue samples removed during surgery. *See also* clinical stage, staging.

percent-free PSA (fPSA): a test that indicates how much prostate-specific antigen (PSA) circulates unbound (alone) in the blood compared to the total amount of PSA. For total PSA results in the borderline range (4 to 10 ng/mL), a low percent free-PSA (25% or less) means that a prostate cancer is more likely to be present and may suggest the need for a biopsy. Also called free-PSA ratio.

pelvic nodes: pelvic lymph nodes; the lymph nodes, located within the pelvis, to which prostate cancer is most likely to spread. These nodes are often removed and examined for cancer (pelvic lymph node dissection) prior to radical prostatectomy.

pelvis: the part of the skeleton that forms a ring of bones in the lower trunk and supports the spine and legs. Cancer may spread (metastasize) to these bones. Pelvis is also used to refer to the general region of the lower trunk surrounded by these bones.

penile implant: an artificial device placed in the penis during surgery to restore erections. *See* prosthesis.

percent-free PSA: *see* free-PSA ratio.

perineum (per-eh-KNEE-um): the area between the anus and the scrotum.

permanent section: a method of preparation of tissue for microscopic examination. The tissue is soaked in formaldehyde, processed in various chemicals, surrounded by a block of wax, sliced very thin, attached to a microscope slide and stained. This process usually takes 1 to 2 days. It provides a clear view of the sample so that the presence or absence of cancer can be determined.

phosphodiesterase (FOS-foh-DI-es-ter-ays) inhibitors: drugs, such as sildenafil (Viagra), that can help men achieve an erection. Not all forms of impotence, however, respond to these drugs.

prognosis (prog-NO-sis): a prediction of the course of disease; the outlook for the chances of survival.

proliferative inflammatory atrophy (PIA): chronic inflammatory prostate lesions that may result in prostate cancer.

prostaglandin (PROS-tuh-GLAN-din) E1: a medicine used to treat impotence in men who have had surgery for treatment of prostate cancer.

ProstaScint™ scan: like the bone scan, the ProstaScint scan uses low-level radioactive material to find cancer that has spread beyond the prostate. But the radioactive material for the ProstaScint scan is attached to an antibody made in a laboratory to recognize and stick to a particular substance. In this case, the antibody sticks to prostate-specific membrane antigen (PSMA), a substance found only in normal and cancerous prostate cells. This test detects spread of prostate cancer to bone as well as lymph nodes and other organs, and that it can clearly distinguish prostate cancer from other cancers and benign disorders. It is most commonly used to look for cancer if the prostate-specific antigen (PSA) level is elevated after treatment.

prostate (PROS-tayt): a gland found only in men. It is located just below the bladder and in front of the rectum. The prostate makes a fluid that is part of semen. The urethra, the tube that carries urine, runs through the prostate.

prostatectomy (PROS-tuh-TEK-toh-mee): surgical removal of all or part of the prostate gland. **Radical prostatectomy** refers to surgery to remove the entire prostate gland, the seminal vesicles, and nearby tissue. A prostatectomy can either be a **perineal prostatectomy** in which the prostate is removed through an incision in the skin between the scrotum and anus or a **retropubic prostatectomy** in which the prostate is removed through an incision in the lower abdomen. A **"nerve sparing" prostatectomy** is a form of radical prostatectomy in which the surgeon attempts to remove the prostate gland but still maintain potency by leaving intact the neurovascular bundles that control erection.

prostate-specific antigen (PSA): a protein made by the prostate gland. Levels of PSA in the blood often go up in men with prostate cancer. The PSA test is used to help find prostate cancer as well as to monitor the results of treatment.

prostate-specific membrane antigen (PSMA): *see* ProstaScint™ scan.

prostatic acid phosphatase (pros-tat-ick a-sid fos-fuh-tace) (PAP): a blood test, like the PSA test, that may be done when looking for evidence of prostate cancer. Unlike the PSA test, the PAP test is not useful for prostate cancer screening. (Note: this is not the same test as the Pap screening test for cervical cancer.) *See also* prostate-specific antigen (PSA).

prostatic intraepithelial neoplasia (prah-STA-tik IN-truh-eh-puh-THEE-lee-ul NEE-oh-PLAY-zhuh) (PIN): a condition in which there are changes in the microscopic appearance of prostate epithelial cells. The condition is not cancer, but it may lead to the development of cancer.

prostatitis (prah-stuh-TY-tis): the inflammation of the prostate, usually the result of an infection. Prostatitis is not cancer.

prosthesis (pros-THEE-sis): an artificial part used to replace or improve the function of a body part. A penile implant is an example of a prosthesis.

proton beam radiation therapy: a technique that uses proton beams instead of conventional radiation to kill or shrink cancer cells. Protons are parts of atoms that cause little damage to tissues they pass through but are very effective in killing cells at the end of their path. This technique may be able to deliver more radiation to the cancer while reducing side effects of nearby normal tissues.

PSA: *see* prostate-specific antigen.

PSA density (PSAD): PSAD is determined by dividing the prostate-specific antigen (PSA) level by the prostate volume (its size as measured by transrectal ultrasound). A higher PSAD indicates greater likelihood of cancer.

PSA doubling time (PSADT): the amount of time it takes for the prostate-specific antigen (PSA) level to double. This measurement is sometimes useful in determining whether cancer is present or has recurred.

PSA velocity (PSAV): a measurement of how quickly the prostate-specific antigen (PSA) level rises over a period of time. This measurement has been suggested as a way to improve the accuracy of PSA testing. A higher PSAV indicates greater likelihood of cancer being present.

rad: stands for "radiation absorbed dose," a measurement of the amount of radiation absorbed by tissues. The term rad is being replaced by cGy (centigray).

radiation therapy (RAY-dee-AY-shun THAYR-uh-pee): treatment with high-energy rays (such as x-rays) to kill or shrink cancer cells. The radiation may come from outside of the body (external radiation) or from radioactive materials placed directly in the tumor (brachytherapy or internal radiation). Radiation therapy may be used as the main treatment for a cancer, to reduce the size of a cancer before surgery, or to destroy any remaining cancer cells after surgery. In advanced cancer cases, it may also be used as palliative treatment. *See also* external beam radiation therapy, brachytherapy, proton beam radiation therapy, rad.

radiopharmaceuticals (RAY-dee-oh-FAR-muh-SOO-tih-kuls): a group of drugs that include radioactive elements, such as strontium-89 or samarium-153, which are given intravenously (IV) to treat bone pain related to metastatic prostate cancer.

rectum: the lower part of the large intestine, just above the anus.

recurrence: the return of cancer after treatment. **Local recurrence** means that the cancer has come back at the same place as the original cancer. **Regional recurrence** means that the cancer has come back after treatment in the lymph nodes near the primary site. **Distant recurrence**, also known as metastatic recurrence, is when cancer metastasizes after treatment to distant organs or tissues (such as the lungs, liver, bone marrow, or brain). *See also* metastasis, metastasize.

regional stage: *see* staging.

remission: complete or partial disappearance of the signs and symptoms of cancer in response to treatment; the period during which a disease is under control. A remission may not be a cure.

resectoscope (reh-SEK-toh-skope): an instrument used in transurethral resection of the prostate (TURP), allowing the surgeon direct inspection of the prostatic urethra and adjacent prostatic tissue.

retropubic (reh-troh-PYOO-bik): behind the pubic bone.

retropubic (reh-troh-PYOO-bik) approach: a surgical approach to the prostate through an incision in the lower abdomen. *See* prostatectomy.

risk factor: anything that affects a person's chance of getting a disease such as cancer. Different cancers have different risk factors. For example, unprotected exposure to strong sunlight is a risk factor for skin cancer; smoking is a risk factor for lung, mouth, larynx, and other cancers. Some risk factors, such as smoking, can be controlled. Others, like a person's age, can't be changed.

saw palmetto: an herbal extract from the berries of the saw palmetto tree that is sometimes used to reduce symptoms of benign prostatic hyperplasia (BPH). It is not a proven treatment for prostate cancer.

screening: the search for disease, such as cancer, in people without symptoms. For example, screening measures for prostate cancer include digital rectal examination and the prostate-specific antigen (PSA) blood test. Screening may refer to coordinated programs in large populations.

scrotum: the pouch of skin that holds the testicles.

selenium (sah-LEEN-e-um): a trace mineral that may play a role in reducing the risk of prostate cancer. Studies are now under way to determine the role of selenium in prostate cancer risk.

semen: fluid released during orgasm; it contains sperm and seminal fluid.

seminal vesicles: glands at the base of the bladder and next to the prostate that release fluid into the semen during orgasm. Cancer that spreads beyond the prostate gland may invade the seminal vesicles.

side effects: unwanted effects of treatment, such as hair loss caused by chemotherapy and fatigue caused by radiation therapy.

sign: an observable physical change caused by an illness. *Compare with* symptom.

stage: the extent of a cancer in the body. *See* staging.

staging: the process of finding out whether cancer has spread and if so, how far. There is more than one system for staging prostate cancer, including the TNM system, the Gleason system, and the Whitmore-Jewett staging system.

The TNM system, which is used most often, gives 3 key pieces of information:

- T refers to the size of the tumor
- N describes how far the cancer has spread to nearby lymph nodes
- M shows whether the cancer has spread (metastasized) to other organs of the body

Letters or numbers after the T, N, and M give more details about each of these factors. To make this information more clear, the TNM descriptions can be grouped together into a simpler set of stages, labeled with Roman numerals (usually from I to IV). In general, the lower the number, the less the cancer has spread. A higher number means a more serious cancer. The 2 types of staging are clinical staging and pathologic staging.

The National Cancer Institute stages cancer in three categories: **Local stage** means the cancer has not invaded the surrounding tissues from the site of origin. **Regional stage** means the cancer has invaded nearby tissues and/ or nearby lymph nodes. **Distant stage** means the cancer has spread to distant parts of the body away from the site of origin. *See also* clinical stage, pathologic stage, Gleason system, Whitmore-Jewett staging system.

stereotactic radiosurgery: a form of radiation therapy that focuses high-powered x-rays on a small area of the body. (With regular radiation therapy, healthy tissue that is nearby also receives radiation.) Stereotactic radiosurgery better focuses the radiation on the abnormal area. Despite its name, it is considered a form of radiation therapy, not a surgical procedure. When many treatments are given, it is called stereotactic radiotherapy.

strontium-89 (Metastron): a radioactive compound that is absorbed by the bone. It is used to treat bone pain associated with prostate cancer. It is injected into a vein and is attracted to areas of bone containing metastatic cancer. The radiation given off by the strontium-89 kills the cancer cells and relieves the pain caused by bone metastases. *See also* radiopharmaceuticals.

symptom: a change in the body caused by an illness, as described by the person experiencing it. *Compare with* sign.

testicles: the male reproductive glands found in the scrotum. The testicles (or testes) produce sperm and the male hormone testosterone.

testosterone (tes-TOS-ter-own): the male hormone, made primarily in the testicles. It stimulates blood flow, growth in certain tissues, and the secondary sexual characteristics. In men with prostate cancer, it can also encourage growth of the tumor.

three-dimensional conformal radiation therapy (3D-CRT): treatment using sophisticated computers to precisely map the location of the cancer within the prostate. The patient is fitted with a plastic mold resembling a body cast to keep him still so that the radiation can be more accurately aimed. Radiation beams are then aimed from several directions. This technique reduces the effects on normal tissues and may allow higher doses of radiation to be used.

tissue: a collection of cells, united to perform a particular function in the body.

transrectal ultrasound (TRUS): an imaging test in which a probe inserted into the rectum gives off sound waves to create a picture of the prostate on a screen to help detect or find the location of tumors.

transurethral resection (TRANZ-yoo-REE-thrul ree-SEK-shun) of the prostate (TURP): an operation that involves removing a part of the prostate gland that surrounds the urethra. The procedure is used for some men with prostate cancer who cannot have a radical prostatectomy because of advanced age or other serious illnesses. This surgical procedure can be used to relieve symptoms caused by a tumor, but it is not expected to cure this disease or remove all of the cancer. TURP is used more often to relieve symptoms of benign prostatic hyperplasia (BPH).

TRUS: *see* transrectal ultrasound.

tumor: an abnormal lump or mass of tissue. Tumors can be benign (noncancerous) or malignant (cancerous).

tumor markers: a substance made by cancer cells and sometimes normal cells. Tumor markers are not very useful for cancer screening because other body tissues not related to a cancer can produce the substance, too. Tumor markers may be very useful in monitoring for response to treatment when a cancer is diagnosed or for a recurrence. Prostate-specific antigen (PSA) is a tumor marker for prostate cancer. *See also* prostate-specific antigen.

tumor suppressor genes: genes that slow down cell division or cause cells to die at the appropriate time. Alterations of these genes can lead to too much cell growth and development of cancer.

TURP: *see* transurethral resection of the prostate.

urethra (yoo-REE-thruh): the tube that carries urine from the bladder outside the body. In women, this tube is fairly short; in men it is longer, passing through the prostate and out through the penis, and it also carries semen. *See also* prostatic urethra; urethral sphincter; urethral stricture.

urethral (yoo-REE-thral) stricture: a narrowing of the urethra due to scar tissue that blocks flow of urine and can result in overflow incontinence. This can be treated by surgically removing the scar tissue and stretching the urethra.

U.S. Food and Drug Administration (FDA): an agency of the United States Department of Health and Human Services. The FDA is responsible for regulating drugs, tobacco products, biological medical products, blood products, medical devices, and radiation-emitting devices, along with other products.

vacuum pump: a device that creates an erection by drawing blood into the penis; a ring placed at the base of the penis traps the blood and sustains the erection.

vas deferens (VAS DEH-feh-RENZ): muscular tubes that carry sperm from the testicles to the urethra.

vasectomy (va-SEK-toh-mee): a surgical procedure in which a segment of each vas deferens is removed to prevent release of sperm and thus provide contraception.

watchful waiting: a form of management of prostate cancer in which the disease is closely monitored (usually with prostate-specific antigen [PSA] blood tests and digital rectal examinations) instead of active treatment such as surgery or radiation therapy. This approach may be a reasonable choice for older men with small tumors that might grow very slowly. If the situation changes, active treatment can be started. Also called expectant management, active surveillance.

Whitmore-Jewett staging system: a classification system for prostate cancer using the categories A, B, C, or D. It has largely been replaced by the TNM system. It can, however, be translated into the TNM system, or the doctor can explain how this staging system will determine treatment options.

x-ray: one form of radiation that can be used at low levels to produce an image of the body on film or at high levels to destroy cancer cells.

Index

Books Published
by the American Cancer Society

Available everywhere books are sold and online at
http://www.cancer.org/bookstore

Information

The American Cancer Society: A History of Saving Lives

American Cancer Society's Complete Guide to Colorectal Cancer

American Cancer Society Complete Guide to Complementary & Alternative Cancer Therapies, Second Edition

American Cancer Society Complete Guide to Nutrition for Cancer Survivors: Eating Well, Staying Well During and After Cancer, Second Edition

Breast Cancer Clear & Simple: All Your Questions Answered

The Cancer Atlas (available in English, Spanish, French, and Chinese)

Cancer: What Causes It, What Doesn't

QuickFACTS™ —Advanced Cancer

QuickFACTS™ —Bone Metastasis

QuickFACTS™ —Colorectal Cancer, Second Edition

QuickFACTS™ —Lung Cancer

QuickFACTS™ —Thyroid Cancer

The Tobacco Atlas, Second Edition (available in English, Spanish, French, and Chinese)

Day-to-Day Help

American Cancer Society's Guide to Pain Control: Understanding and Managing Cancer Pain, Revised Edition

Cancer Caregiving A to Z: An At-Home Guide for Patients and Families

Caregiving: A Step-By-Step Resource for Caring for the Person with Cancer at Home, Revised Edition

Get Better! Communication Cards for Kids & Adults

Kicking Butts: Quit Smoking and Take Charge of Your Health, Second Edition

Lymphedema: Understanding and Managing Lymphedema After Cancer Treatment

Social Work in Oncology: Supporting Survivors, Families and Caregivers

What to Eat During Cancer Treatment

When the Focus Is on Care: Palliative Care and Cancer

Emotional Support

Angels & Monsters: A child's eye view of cancer

Cancer in the Family: Helping Children Cope with a Parent's Illness

Chemo and Me: My Hair Loss Experience

Couples Confronting Cancer: Keeping Your Relationship Strong

Crossing Divides: A Couple's Story of Cancer, Hope, and Hiking Montana's Continental Divide

I Can Survive

The Survivorship Net: A Parable for the Family, Friends, and Caregivers of People with Cancer

What Helped Get Me Through: Cancer Survivors Share Wisdom and Hope

Just for Kids

Because . . . Someone I Love Has Cancer: Kids' Activity Book

Healthy Me: A Read-Along Coloring & Activity Book

Jacob Has Cancer: His Friends Want to Help

Kids' First Cookbook: Delicious-Nutritious Treats To Make Yourself!

Let My Colors Out

Mom and the Polka-Dot Boo-Boo

Nana, What's Cancer?

No Thanks, but I'd Love to Dance

Our Dad Is Getting Better

Our Mom Has Cancer (hardcover)

Our Mom Has Cancer (paperback)

Our Mom Is Getting Better

What's Up with Bridget's Mom? Medikidz Explain Breast Cancer

What's Up with Richard? Medikidz Explain Leukemia

Prevention

The American Cancer Society's Healthy Eating Cookbook: A celebration of food, friendship, and healthy living, Third Edition

Celebrate! Healthy Entertaining for Any Occasion

Good for You! Reducing Your Risk of Developing Cancer

The Great American Eat-Right Cookbook: 140 Great-Tasting, Good-for-You Recipes

Healthy Air: A Read-Along Coloring & Activity Book
(25 per pack: Tobacco avoidance)

Healthy Bodies: A Read-Along Coloring & Activity Book
(25 per pack: Physical activity)

Healthy Food: A Read-Along Coloring & Activity Book
(25 per pack: Nutrition)

National Health Education Standards: Achieving Excellence, Second Edition (available in paperback and on CD-ROM)

Reduce Your Cancer Risk